Care of the Neur

I

Care of the
Neurological Patient

Helen Iggulden
BA (Hons), MSc, RGN, RNT
Lecturer in Nursing
University of Salford

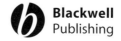

© 2006 H. Iggulden
Blackwell Publishing Ltd
Editorial offices:
Blackwell Publishing Ltd, 9600 Garsington Road, Oxford OX4 2DQ, UK
    Tel: +44 (0)1865 776868
Blackwell Publishing Inc., 350 Main Street, Malden, MA 02148-5020, USA
    Tel: +1 781 388 8250
Blackwell Publishing Asia Pty Ltd, 550 Swanston Street, Carlton, Victoria
3053, Australia
    Tel: +61 (0)3 8359 1011

First published 2006 by Blackwell Publishing Ltd

ISBN-13: 978-14051-1716-6
ISBN-10: 1-4051-1716-8

Library of Congress Cataloging-in-Publication Data
Iggulden, Helen.
  Care of the neurological patient / Helen Iggulden.
      p. ; cm.
  Includes bibliographical references and index.
  ISBN-13: 978-1-4051-1716-6 (pbk. : alk. paper)
  ISBN-10: 1-4051-1716-8 (pbk. : alk. paper)
  1. Neurological nursing. 2. Nervous system–Diseases–Patients–Care.
I. Title.
  [DNLM: 1. Nervous System Diseases–nursing. 2. Activities of Daily
Living. 3. Evidence–Based Medicine.   WY 160.5 I24c 2006]
RC350.5.I33 2006
616.8′04231–dc22

2005025427

A catalogue record for this title is available from the British Library

Set in 9 on 11pt Palatino
by SNP Best-set Typesetter Ltd., Hong Kong
Printed and bound in Singapore
by COS Printer

The publisher's policy is to use permanent paper from mills that operate a
sustainable forestry policy, and which has been manufactured from pulp
processed using acid-free and elementary chlorine-free practices.
Furthermore, the publisher ensures that the text paper and cover board
used have met acceptable environmental accreditation standards.

For further information on Blackwell Publishing, visit our website:
www.blackwellnursing.com

Contents

Foreword   vi
Preface and Definition of Terms   viii
Acknowledgements   xii
How to Use this Book   xiii
Glossary of Neurological Conditions and Terms   xviii

1 Background Anatomy and Physiology   1
2 Nursing Assessment   28
3 Maintaining a Safe Environment   52
4 Communicating   86
5 Breathing   105
6 Eating and Drinking   124
7 Eliminating   153
8 Washing and Dressing   176
9 Controlling Body Temperature   191
10 Mobilising   201
11 Working and Playing   229
12 Expressing Sexuality   248
13 Sleeping   257
14 Dying   272
15 National Service Framework for Long Term Conditions
and Skill Competencies in Neurological Care   289

Appendix 1   Resources and Support Groups   294
Appendix 2   Further Reading   301
Index   303

Foreword

More than 10 million people in the UK are affected by a neurological disorder and over 18 000 cases of major disability might be prevented simply by improved recognition of warning signs by patients and their doctors – it is a frightening statistic against a backdrop of low recognition for the speciality of neurology. Caring for patients with neurological conditions is both challenging and rewarding and requires special skills and knowledge. The continuing problems faced by healthcare systems today mean that staff are constantly juggling the resources to meet an ever increasing demand on services, therefore the knowledge and skills of the neurological nurse become crucial in the management of the patient and their family.

The Long-term Conditions National Service Framework, launched in March 2005, aims to transform the way health and social care services support people to live with long-term neurological conditions. The key themes are: independent living; care planned around the needs and choices of the individual; easier, timely access to services; and joint working across all agencies and disciplines involved. These principles fit neatly with the management of neurological conditions and are identified in this book.

This book fills an identified gap to describe the care of the neurological patient. It has the potential to meet the main objective of a 'return to the basics of nursing care', which appears to have been forgotten in the ever increasing technological world we find ourselves in today. The text is organised in a logical fashion so that units can be studied as relevant to patient care and care may be planned and reasoned accordingly.

The presentation is innovative and genuinely able to offer a new and worthwhile activity to all levels of staff, and emphasises the multidisciplinary nature of patient care in this patient group. Therefore, the aim has to be to improve the quality of life for people affected by neurological conditions in the specialist or generalist setting.

Whether a novice or an expert in the field of neurology, whether working in a specialist environment, a general ward or community setting, this text offers something for all levels of staff. Many patients with neurological conditions are cared for in general hospitals or the community and not in major teaching hospitals, so this text will truly add value to a diverse staff group. Those who study this text as applied to their clinical practice should then be able to develop the capacity and skill with which to plan and deliver care for the neurological patient to the highest quality standards.

This text is a key tool for understanding and delivering the care to support people with neurological and long-term conditions. By heightening awareness of the impact of neurological conditions, the importance of attention to detail and concentrating on the fundamentals of care, it is an exciting development to promote the dissemination of information about neurological conditions to a wider healthcare audience and to ensure that those affected are involved in the management of their condition.

By securing the highest standards of service and improved care for people with neurological conditions, regardless of the environment, outcomes for patients and their families should be improved.

Elizabeth A. Preston, January 2006

Preface

Although more than 8 million people in Britain are affected by a neurological condition, the vast majority are able to manage the everyday tasks of their lives. However, more than 1 million people are disabled by their condition and about 350 000 require help for most of their daily activities.

Many of these people will be nursed outside specialist units; in fact, Morrow and Patterson (1997) estimate that acute neurology cases account for 20% of admissions to general medical wards and would be looked after by general nurses. The need for these nurses to understand the care of the neurological patient has been recognised by new benchmarks which were created in March 2005. The National Service Framework for Long Term Conditions created 11 quality-based standards to help deliver and integrate services in a general and specialist setting. The new standards should also support the needs of the individual in acute, rehabilitation and lifelong care.

In the light of the new requirements, this book will be a useful and practical resource both for nurses and students working in non-specialist areas and for those new to a specialist setting. For deeper understanding of neurological conditions, the book should be used in conjunction with more detailed specialist texts.

Guidance will be given for the care of patients after acquired brain injury such as stroke or sub-arachnoid haemorrhage; traumatic injury or anoxic damage; seizure activity; dementia; multiple sclerosis; Parkinson's disease; and motor neurone disease. The book is succinct in style and focuses on the problems and discomforts that patients commonly experience. It will outline the clinical skills used most often and most effectively to respond to patients' needs.

For clarity and brevity, patients' problems are set out using the Roper–Logan–Tierney 'twelve activities for living', and are not associated with a specific disease. The 'activities for living' nursing model includes the following: maintaining a safe environment; communicating; breathing; eating and drinking; eliminating; personal cleansing and dressing; controlling body temperature; mobilising; working and playing; expressing sexuality; sleeping; and dying.

Most nurses in the UK are familiar with this model and its holistic philosophy, which takes into account biological, psychological, socio-cultural and politico-economic factors in developing individualised care. It is assumed that readers are familiar with this model. Anyone unfamiliar with the 12 activities should consult Holland *et al.* (2003) and explore the different dimensions of the model through a variety of case studies and exercises.

Some background anatomy and physiology will be given where it is essential to understanding common problems such as pain, falling, confusion, swallowing difficulties, breathing difficulties, fatigue, communication and elimination problems, sitting and walking balance, sexual dysfunction, and perceptual and cognitive disturbances that affect work and leisure activity.

This textbook suggests that all patients' difficulties, problems or needs should be seen in relation to one, some or all of the following: altered sensation, altered movement or motor ability, altered perception, and altered cognition, which can occur to some extent in almost any neurological disease. The following terms are used to describe our awareness and function.

DEFINITION OF TERMS

Sensation. The ability of the sensory nerves to pick up and conduct information relating to touch, temperature, pressure, pain, equilibrium and position, and the special senses involving hearing, sight, smell and taste.

Altered sensation. Caused by damage to the nerves picking up sensation. It may be experienced as pins and needles, numbness, tingling, hypersensitivity or hyposensitivity to temperature, pressure or pain, or as disturbances of visual acuity, balance and equilibrium.

Perception. The ability of the sensory area of the brain to identify, interpret and attach meaning to incoming sensory information using both sensory stimulation and reason.

Altered perception. Usually caused by brain damage affecting this sensory area. It can affect accuracy and ability in recognising colour, depth, figure and background, shape and form, face recognition, constructional ability, body image, and schema and route finding.

Cognition. Works hand in hand with perceptual processing using attention, orientation, concentration, short- and long-term memory, storage and retrieval, problem solving, decision making, planning, organising, reasoning, concept forming, goal formation and error detection.

Altered cognition. Most commonly seen in brain injury, dementia and other neuro-degenerative conditions. It may manifest as insufficient alertness, distractability, lack of concentration, slowed information processing, inability to organise and sequence tasks, impaired memory, impaired judgement of personal safety, low frustration tolerance, lack of insight, poor behavioural control.

Movement or motor ability. The ability to initiate and sustain co-ordinated muscle activity to maintain and modify body function, posture, position and the position of the limbs and body parts in relation to each other and the outside world.

Altered motor ability. Most commonly evident as muscle paralysis, weakness, fatigue or excess activity such as rigidity or spasticity caused by damage to the motor nerves locally or in the motor pathways of the brain itself.

Mood and emotion. Can be affected by damage or disease in the nervous system either as a direct result of the altered physiology or because of perceptual and cognitive appraisal of the situation in which people find themselves. Moods and emotions are usually categorised as positive or negative and can affect sensation, perception, cognition and motor ability positively or negatively.

REFERENCES

Holland, K., Jenkins, J., Solomon, J. and Whittam, S. (2003) *Applying the Roper Logan and Tierney Model in Practice.* Churchill Livingstone, Edinburgh.

Morrow, J. and Patterson, V. (1997) The neurological practice of a district general hospital. *Journal of Neurology, Neurosurgery and Psychiatry* **63** (Supplement), S39–S52.

Acknowledgements

For their invaluable specialist knowledge in helping to develop the case studies I am grateful to Janet Comer, Carole Cromwell, Michelle Devine, Dawn Gawthorpe, Fran Jackson, Sam Holden-Smith, Colette Manning, Sarah Nicholson, Steve Pymm and Krystyna Walton.

For help in reviewing the drafts and providing invaluable comments I am grateful to Beth Knight and Katharine Taylor.

I am very grateful to all publishers who have given their kind permission to reproduce material from their publications.

How to Use this Book

Information is condensed as far as possible through frequent use of sub-headings, lists, bullet points, figures, boxes and tables. The references and suggested further reading provide ideas for more detailed material.

The information given in each chapter is illustrated and discussed through one or more case studies, which are outlined in the following pages. These scenarios are referred to in the main text to show how care planning can be reasoned and applied to practice. However, this textbook could also be used without the case studies and fuller discussion, serving as a quick reference guide to the appropriate course of action. The glossary gives an outline of the main neurological conditions covered.

CASE STUDIES

1. Harry

Harry is a 72-year-old man who suffered a brain haemorrhage several weeks ago while out at the market doing his Saturday shopping. He has spent a lot of the time sleeping but now seems to be waking up. He is restless in bed though, constantly rubbing his legs against the sheets in repetitive movements. Sometimes he also plucks at the sheets and tries to rearrange them. When he does get out of bed or up out of the chair, he does not seem to know where he is or why he has got up. Sometimes he says he wants to go to the toilet, and sometimes he has become abusive, demanding to go home. As the ward is short of staff to supervise him one-to-one, the possibility of sedation is being considered.

After being on the ward for a few days, Harry's behaviour changes and becomes unpredictable. Sometimes he sleeps like a log all night and is very difficult to rouse in the morning. At other times he seems to sleep very little at night, he is extremely restless, he makes a lot of noises and shouts out although he does not use comprehensible words, and he often gets up and wanders about.

After being on the ward for a few days he starts to touch female staff in a sexually suggestive way. Unsure of how to deal with situation, they start to avoid contact with him and his care is being compromised.

2. Mark

Mark is in his twenties and was involved in a fight outside a nightclub three weeks ago. He was taken to the accident and emergency department of a district general hospital and transferred to a neurosurgical specialist unit when his Glasgow Coma Scale (GCS) became 10. After two weeks he was transferred to a general surgical ward as there were more acutely ill patients needing specialist help. Although reasonably stable he still seems to spend a long time sleeping. The nurse who accompanies him tells the receiving nurse that his neurological observations have been reduced to daily, but she is unable to provide information about his condition or treatment as she is an agency nurse. The receiving nurse notices that while sitting, Mark lolls to one side, that he is drooling, and when he gets up to walk across to his bed, his gait is unsteady, uneven and he bumps into the furniture. As Mark recovers he develops an insatiable appetite. He asks for food persistently throughout the day, and when he eats he bolts his food down.

3. Irene

Irene had been experiencing weakness in her lower limbs and slight slurring of speech for several weeks before contacting her GP who referred her to the nearest general hospital for further investigations. As a result of the investigations, she is diagnosed as having motor neurone disease. She managed well in the community for a couple of months, with the support of her 70-year-old partner Bob, a community physiotherapist, an occupational therapist, a speech and language therapist, and check-up appointments in outpatients. Recently however she has been admitted to a hospital providing specialist neurological services because she has started experiencing shortness of breath, morning headaches, increased sleepiness during the day, and restless nights.

4. Miriam

Miriam is in her early sixties and had a sub-arachnoid haemor-rhage six weeks ago. She had a tracheostomy and was unwell for some time. She has now been transferred from the high dependency unit to a general medical ward having had her tracheostomy removed five days ago. She has had a percutaneous endoscopic gastrostomy (PEG) tube inserted but now needs to start feeding orally. Videofluoroscopy and assessment by a speech and language therapist indicate that she can begin to take thickened fluids and puréed food orally. She is reluctant to eat, however, and although she has the motor ability to use utensils she is leaving her food untouched.

5. Louise

Louise is 32 and has had multiple sclerosis for the past four years. She has two children aged 5 and 7 years and her husband works long hours as a lorry driver. She has recently had a relapse, feeling a burning sensation in her legs, and she feels that the left leg particularly is weaker and that she is getting more fatigued more easily. She is also having difficulty passing water and has abdominal pain although reduced perianal sensation. She tells you that recently things have been getting 'on top of' her, that she is not sleeping well and is feeling quite down, and that she has been smoking a lot more than usual. She is also worried about her relationship with her husband, particularly as she seems to have lost interest in the sexual side of it, mostly, she thinks, because of the loss of sensation.

6. Anwah

Two years ago Anwah, a 32-year-old mother of three children, suffered meningitis. She was ventilated, had a tracheostomy performed and was nursed in intensive care for two months. She was successfully weaned from the ventilator and has been transferred to a general medical ward, but still has her tracheostomy from which she coughs copious loose secretions.

She does not speak but makes eye contact and smiles, laughs and cries. She is fed by percutaneous endoscopic gastrostomy tube. She cannot maintain a sitting position unaided, but can grasp objects with her hands. The ward she has come from did not have suitable facilities for bathing or showering her and she seems apprehensive when she thinks she is going to have a wash. Nursing staff think she is frightened because she wails and her whole body tone increases when they approach her in the morning to help her wash.

7. Gary

Three weeks ago Gary was struck by a car while he was getting out of a taxi. He sustained a head injury for which he has received treatment in a neurosurgical unit. He has been transferred to a general hospital ward until a neurorehabilitation bed becomes available. He has difficulty supporting his head and neck and his head hangs forward when he is sitting up. He has poor sitting balance and is unstable when sitting on the side of the bed. When he walks he is unsteady, keeping his legs stiff. His right arm is bent upwards and across his body, and his left arm extends out to the side to try to help him keep his balance.

8. Joyce

Joyce was involved in a road accident in Spain and was nursed there until she was well enough to return to the UK by air ambulance. She is admitted to a rehabilitation ward for assessment and is referred to the acute medical team as she has a severe chest infection. She also has severe painful spasticity in both legs, complicated by an arthitic left knee which she had before the accident. Because her legs are so tightly flexed, nursing staff are finding it difficult to help her with her elimination and hygiene needs. This tightness is also interfering with her progress, levels of independence and other activities. Although she is currently on oral baclofen, this drug does not seem to be effective. She has dysarthria, her speech is slow and unclear but she uses eye pointing and a light writer effectively. She has some swallowing difficulty and needs thickened fluids and a soft diet.

9. Fred

Fred is 72 years old and has suffered from Parkinson's disease for the past eight years. He lives at home with his 70-year-old wife who is his main carer. He has a son and a daughter but neither live near home. He has been admitted to a neuromedical ward via his GP because he is experiencing hallucinations and frequent 'on' and 'off' periods. His wife has been finding it difficult to cope and he has become very reluctant to let her manage his medication.

10. Ella

Ella is in her mid-forties and has worked night shifts as a nursing assistant at her local hospital for the past ten years. She collapsed while at work a week ago and was admitted to the medical ward. It has been established that she has suffered cerebrovascular accident. She has a very dense right hemiplegia, dysphasia and swallowing problems. She is a large lady weighing 18 stone, she cries a lot, winces and wails, which sound very much as if she is in pain. The physiotherapist cannot detect signs of spasticity and thinks that she may be suffering from 'central pain'. She attends to what is being said to her, is able to nod and shake her head appropriately, and has facial expressions indicating puzzlement, surprise, annoyance and pleasure. She can recognise familiar objects such as a bar of soap and a face flannel. However, she is not able to follow directions by language alone, has not yet used the call bell, and is not able to write or recognise her name. She sometimes says odd phrases such as 'get the bath thing', but this does not seem to indicate that she wants a bath.

Glossary of Neurological Conditions and Terms

Agnosia. A perceptual disorder in which a person cannot identify an object despite the ability to recognise its tactile and visual elements.

Aphasia. May also be called dysphasia. The impaired ability to understand and/or produce spoken and written language, which may extend to other forms of symbolic representation such as visual symbols differentiating male and female toilets.

Apraxia. Where the person is unable to carry out purposeful, previously learned motor acts despite physical ability, willingness and an understanding of an instruction such as 'raise your right hand'.

Articulation. The sound and pitch of the tone emerging from the larynx is converted by movements of the tongue, soft palate and lips to speech

Articulatory dyspraxia, oral apraxia. The loss of the ability to carry out skilled movements, and, although not technically a language-processing problem, it causes loss of the ability to co-ordinate tongue, cheek and lip movements to produce speech.

Ataxia. Incoordination caused by damage to the cerebellum or the sensory pathways that convey information about the position of joints; manifests as abnormal gait or arm movements.

Contracture. Permanent fibrosis of soft tissue and muscle around a joint that fixes a limb in flexion.

Critical-illness neuropathy. Can develop in up to 50% of patients who have been in a critical care unit for more than two weeks. There may be marked weakness of respiratory muscles, sensory loss and weakness. Time, good nutrition and hydration, and a period of care will usually ensure a good recovery.

Dermatome. An area of skin that has its sensation from a single nerve via single nerve root in the spinal cord.

Electrolyte. Any substance that, in solution, will conduct an electric current. Electrolytes affect the movement of substances between body fluids and tissues. In the generation of an action potential following a stimulus, the electrolytes involved in nerve conduction are sodium and potassium.

Enteral nutrition. Refers to nutrition support delivered through a tube to the stomach, duodenum or jejunum.

Epilepsy. Also known as a seizure disorder. Epilepsy is usually diagnosed after someone has experienced at least two seizures. Most of the time the cause is unknown, although it may be related to brain injury or family tendency. A seizure is a sudden surge of electrical activity in the brain that originates from many different brain disorders. This surge of activity may be barely noticeable to others or it may involve loss of consciousness and motor control for a short time. If a seizure originates in a specific area of the brain then the initial symptoms of the seizure often reflect the functions of that area, so seizures may take many forms. A good history of what the triggers are and a comprehensive seizure activity record will facilitate accurate diagnosis and ensure seizure control with minimal side effects. Further information from Epilepsy Action at http://www.epilepsy.org.uk

Fluency. The term used to describe smooth, rapid, effortless use of language.

Guillain-Barré syndrome (GBS). An acute inflammation of the nerves of the peripheral nervous system that causes sudden weakness and limb paralysis and a loss of sensation sometimes with pain. It is thought that an infection in the preceding few weeks may trigger a reaction in the immune system, which attacks the nerves. It usually begins with tingling or numbness in the fingers and toes, with progressive weakness in the arms and legs over the next few days. It may remain mild, but can progress to complete paralysis of the legs, and may even progress up the chest, paralysing the muscles of breathing so that mechanical ventilation is required. The throat and face may also be affected, leading to impaired swallowing and the need for tube feeding through the stomach. Recovery usually occurs spontaneously, with good medicine, nursing and physiotherapy. Further details can be obtained from the GBS Support Group at http://gbs.org.uk

Intonation. The different levels of pitch or tone that are used in particular sequences to express a wide range of meaning.

Meningitis. The inflammation of the lining around the brain and spinal cord caused by bacteria or virus. It begins with a stiff neck, severe headache, dislike of bright lights, fever, vomiting, feeling drowsy and the appearance of a rash. It can be fatal in hours, but most people survive although there may be physical and emotional after-effects, ranging from mild to severe depending on the severity of the illness. These after-effects can include memory and concentration impairments, co-ordination problems, headache, deafness, cognitive impairment, seizures, weakness, paralysis and spasticity, speech problems or visual problems. Further information is available from the Meningitis Research Foundation at http://www.meningitis.org

Motor neurone disease. A degenerative disease of upper and lower motor neurones in the brain and spinal cord which leads to weakness and wasting of muscles. Its cause is still being researched. The disease can affect voluntary control of the arms and legs, with some muscle groups being affected more than others. Innervation of the muscles supporting the head, neck and trunk is disturbed causing weakness, with involvement of the muscles of speech, swallowing and breathing. Because only motor nerves are affected there is no loss of sensation or intelligence, perception or awareness. The progress of the disease is unpredictable, and may be very rapid or may take place slowly over many years. Further details are available from the Motor Neurone Disease Association (MNDA) at http://mndassociation.org/full-site/home

Motor restlessness and repetitive movements. Some types of neurological impairment result in restless, repetitive and purposeless movements which can lead to shearing or friction damage to the skin

Multiple sclerosis (MS). MS is caused by the breakdown of myelin, a substance that is wrapped around many neurones both to protect them and to insulate them so speeding up the conduction of electrical impulses. This breakdown is thought to be caused by an autoimmune condition that mistakes the myelin for a foreign body and attacks it. The myelin becomes scarred, and nerve conduction is interrupted, slowed down, distorted or prevented entirely. Both sensory and motor nerves can be affected. Tiredness or fatigue is a very common symptom, as are muscle stiffness and spasms, and there are often sensory disturbances such as tingling, numbness, painful hypersensitivity, slurred speech, and blurred or double vision. There may also be disturbances of bladder, bowel and sexual function. In addition, MS can be responsible for forgetfulness, difficulty in concentrating, mood swings and depression. There are different types of MS, of which the most common is relapsing–remitting. This means that the person experiences attacks followed by periods of remission that may last for months or years. A progressive form worsens from onset; a relapsing type may develop a progressive pattern. MS cannot be cured but many symptoms such as bladder dysfunction, constipation, depression, fatigue, spasticity, tremor and frequency can be helped by medication and symptom management, and flare-ups will usually respond to steroid therapy. Helpful detailed information is available from the Multiple Sclerosis Society at http://www.mssociety.org.uk

Neurogenic bladder. Term used to describe problems of bladder storage or voiding that are caused by impaired nerve function.

Neuropathy. Inflammation or degeneration of peripheral nerves leading to loss of function and abnormal sensation.

Parkinson's disease. Caused by loss of nerve cells in the substantia nigra of the brain that produces the neurotransmitter dopamine. This substance is responsible for initiating activity in the motor pathways that stimulate the co-ordinated muscle activity needed for any movement. This lack of dopamine causes hesitancy, tremor, stiffness and rigidity when the person wants get up, walk or make some other movement, and sometimes the person fails to initiate a movement at all. Although there is no cure for Parkinson's disease, a number of medications can help manage the symptoms. These include replacing the missing dopamine, for which levodopa is the mainstay and first line of treatment. While the dose is being established, the patient may experience 'on' periods of reasonably fluid movement and 'off' periods of very slowed movement. For a time the established dose may work well, but as further nerve cells degenerate the dose may need to be increased, and this may bring side effects such as dyskinesias. These are unplanned writhing movements of the limbs, trunk or face. Eventually the side effects may be so troublesome that other susbstitute medications need to be used. Helpful and detailed information on the disease, its management and support is available form the Parkinson's Disease Society at http://www.parkinsons.org.uk

Phonation. Refers to the sound produced from the larynx.

Proprioceptors. Special receptors located in muscles and tendons that carry messages to the brain about where the limb is in relation to the body. Patients with loss of proprioception may be unaware that a limb is dangling, that they are lying on it or that it is trapped in an awkward position.

Spasticity. Increased tone in muscles because of damage to upper motor neurones, causing pain, cramps and inability to carry out a movement smoothly.

Stroke. Usually caused by part of the brain being deprived of its blood supply by a blood clot, with resulting cell death. The effect this has on a person depends on both the size of the clot and where in the brain the clot is situated. The commonest symptoms include weakness, paralysis or numbness on one side of the body, visual disturbance, difficulty understanding and producing speech, problems with balance, feeling dizzy, difficulty with bowel and bladder control, depression, problems with perception and cognition, disturbed sensation and fatigue. Treatment is symptomatic and current guidelines recommend early anti-thrombolytic therapy to reduce secondary effects. Other treatments aim to control spasms, pain, depression and prevent further clots forming. The early involvement of the multidisciplinary team is essential. Further details from the Stroke Association at http://www.stroke.org.uk

Sub-arachnoid haemorrhage. Caused by the rupture of blood vessels in the space between the middle membrane (the arachnoid mater) and the inner membrane (the pia mater). The patient usually complains of a severe headache, feeling sick and sleepy or losing consciousness, experiencing seizure activity and confusion. The treatment often involves complex brain surgery to remove an aneurysm or to place a small metal coil at its centre to prevent re-bleeding. Epileptic seizures may occur at any time in the following 12 to 24 months. In addition, stroke may complicate recovery, and the drug nimodipine may be used for the first few weeks after haemorrhage to reduce the risk of a stroke occurring. There may be periods of vasospasm causing transient, even fleeting, changes in consciousness, activity and pain experience. Other post-operative problems may include difficulty opening the jaw, headaches, and numbness round the scar. Drugs to reduce the risk of contraction of blood vessels leading to stroke, to control fits and to lower blood pressure may be needed. Further details can be found at the Brain and Spinal Injury Charity at http://www.basiccharity.org.uk

Background Anatomy and Physiology **1**

INTRODUCTION

The principal concepts of sensation, perception, cognition and movement, which have already been explained in the Preface, provide us with a simple framework for neurological assessment and care planning. This chapter uses that framework to outline the bodily structure and function of the nervous system. It also gives enough depth and detail to provide the essential information that underpins a reasoned approach to nursing assessment and care planning. The number of anatomical terms used is kept to a minimum in order to maintain focus on the concepts and processes involved. However, it is necessary to include a straightforward outline of how receptor stimulation causes signals along nerve pathways and how these signals are transmitted to the spine and brain to initiate movement through the motor pathways. A brief mention is also made of the higher-level functions of perception and cognition.

This chapter also uses the case studies which are set out in the section on How to Use this Book. These illustrate how some conditions affect people physically, cognitively, emotionally and psychologically. In this chapter these include multiple sclerosis, Parkinson's disease, epilepsy, cerebrovascular accident, motor neurone disease and traumatic brain injury.

LEARNING OUTCOMES

- ❏ Understand the overall structure and functioning units of the brain, spinal cord and peripheral nervous system.
- ❏ Understand how damage or disease in these structures can cause altered sensation, altered motor ability or altered perception and cognition.
- ❏ Appreciate how this background information can provide a rationale for assessment and care planning.

OVERVIEW OF THE NERVOUS SYSTEM

For the purposes of study, Figure 1.1 shows a simplified structure of the nervous system, which is often divided for convenience into two parts. It is important to remember, however, that the division *is* convenient, and that the two main parts actually interact dynamically.

- The *central nervous system* consists of the brain and the spinal cord. The spine analyses sensory information and initiates a reflex motor response. The lower brain stimulates homeostatic mechanisms. The cortex analyses complex information and initiates reasoned action.
- The *peripheral nervous system* is made up of 12 pairs of cranial nerves which connect to the brain and 31 pairs of spinal nerves which connect to the spinal cord (see Figure 1.1).

The nerve tissue that makes up the brain and spinal cord develops from a neural tube in the human embryo. As the embryo develops, the neural tube differentiates to form functional regions called the higher brain, midbrain, lower brain and spinal cord (see Figure 1.2). The functions of the system are either voluntary or involuntary. The voluntary function regulates the muscles that we use to stand, run, raise an arm or generally move. The involuntary or autonomic function regulates body homeostasis, such as heart rate, breathing rate or hormone secretion, thirst, appetite, body temperature and so on. The main difference between autonomic and other nerves is the kind of tissue that the nerve contacts. The autonomic (involuntary) nerves

- contact glands and internal organs, and
- regulate activities such as the heart rate, sweating, stomach contractions and the size of the pupil of the eye (see Figure 1.3).

By contrast, the somatic (voluntary) nerves

- contact skeletal muscle, and
- regulate voluntary movement.

Both the central and peripheral parts of the system are made up of *neurones* that form *pathways*. Sensory information such as temperature, touch, pain, vision and smell is carried to the brain

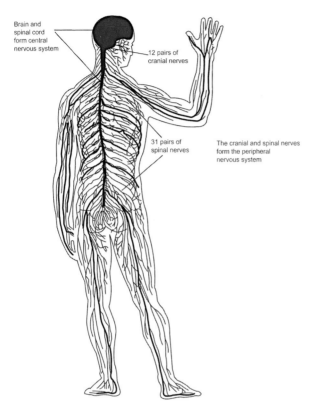

Brain and
spinal cord
form central
nervous system

12 pairs of
cranial nerves

31 pairs of
spinal nerves

The cranial and spinal nerves
form the peripheral
nervous system

Figure 1.1 Nerveman showing overall organisation of the brain, spinal cord and peripheral nervous system.

and spinal cord through sensory pathways. Once the stimulus is analysed, at either a conscious or an unconscious level, motor pathways generate a motor response. Neurological observations, particularly the *Glasgow Coma Scale*, estimate the level at which the patient is responding – from the peripheral, spinal or lower brain level or higher brain. Sensory or motor signals are generated at the end of a neurone by the release of a substance

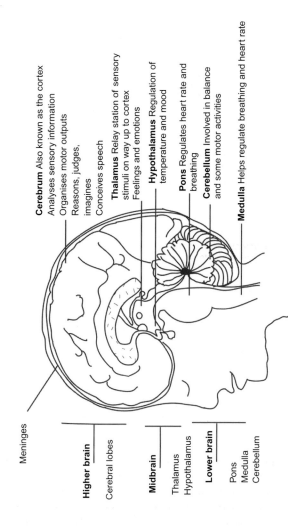

Cerebrum Also known as the cortex
Analyses sensory information
Organises motor outputs
Reasons, judges,
imagines
Conceives speech

Thalamus Relay station of sensory
stimuli on way up to cortex
Feelings and emotions

Hypothalamus Regulation of
temperature and mood

Pons Regulates heart rate and
breathing

Cerebellum Involved in balance
and some motor activities

Medulla Helps regulate breathing and heart rate

Meninges

Higher brain

Cerebral lobes

Midbrain

Thalamus
Hypothalamus

Lower brain

Pons
Medulla
Cerebellum

Figure 1.2 The functions of higher brain, midbrain and lower brain.

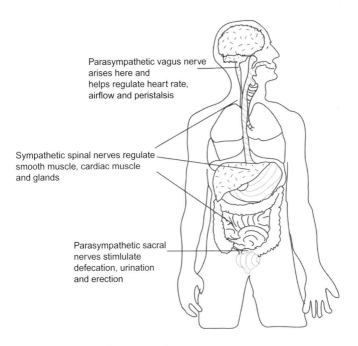

Parasympathetic vagus nerve arises here and helps regulate heart rate, airflow and peristalsis

Sympathetic spinal nerves regulate smooth muscle, cardiac muscle and glands

Parasympathetic sacral nerves stimlulate defecation, urination and erection

Figure 1.3 Functions of the autonomic nerves.

called a *neurotransmitter*. These substances generate electrical impulses in other nerves or stimulate contraction of a muscle.

An analogy

It may help to visualise this nerve network as a railway network. You can imagine London as the central system and other main cities north of London forming the peripheral system. Southbound trains, or sensory nerves, carry sensory information to several main stations in London, which in the analogy represents the brain and spinal cord. Northbound trains, or motor nerves, carry motor instructions out to the peripheral cities, which correspond to the cranial and spinal nerves. Smaller and smaller divisions of these nerves, just like local rail networks to small towns and villages, carry messages on to the muscles and skin.

Imagine that the rail tracks are pathways made up of neurones and that the train signals of stop or go are the neurotransmitters that control whether or not a train moves. Imagine that the train itself is the nerve impulse, carrying its electrical message along the track, to arrive at the correct destination, on time, with no diversions. To achieve this, there should be no broken rail tracks, which represent damage to the continuity of the pathways, no mechanical failure of the train, which represents electrical faults that prevent the impulse from travelling through the neurone, and no faulty signals, which can be seen as the failure of a neurotransmitter to prevent or stimulate action.

The main purpose of the nerve network is to keep us safe and well, by allowing unimpeded sensation to give us information upon which we act – for example, telling us when we are too hot, too cold or too sleepy for comfort. The nerve networks carry messages about external and internal sensations from the peripheral nerves to the spinal cord and to the brain. The brain analyses the sensory information and registers a pleasurable or unpleasurable feeling. It then produces signals that travel down the spine from the brain and out to the peripheral nerves. These then stimulate muscle movement. These movements may be voluntary or involuntary.

Voluntary and involuntary movement and reflexes
Voluntary movement is usually initiated from a higher region of the brain, called the cortex, which stimulates skeletal muscle. *Involuntary movement* is initiated much lower down in the lower brain and brain stem, and maintains tone in the smooth muscles needed to co-ordinate heart rate, breathing and other homeostatic functions. *Reflexes* are initiated from the spinal cord and sensory information may need not travel up as far as the brain to generate a motor response.

Neurones
Nerves are made up of bundles of neurones. The three main parts of a neurone or nerve cell are *dendrites*, a *cell body* and an

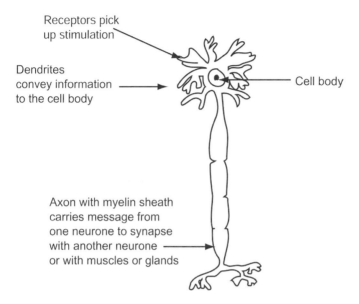

Receptors pick up stimulation

Dendrites convey information to the cell body

Cell body

Axon with myelin sheath carries message from one neurone to synapse with another neurone or with muscles or glands

Figure 1.4 Outline of neurone.

axon (see Figure 1.4). Specialised *receptors* on the end of the dendrites pick up sensations such as touch or temperature. The dendrites pick up stimulation and the axons convey stimulation to another neurone. The receptors stimulate the dendrites, which then send a message electrically towards the cell.

Conduction of electrical message along a neurone

A message is conducted along the neurone by the action of the *electrolytes* (sodium and potassium) across its membrane. The neurone is like a mini battery with a negative charge on the inside separated from a positive charge on the outside by a membrane.

When at rest, the membrane normally allows the passage of potassium out of the cell while preventing sodium entering the cell. This is called the *resting potential*. When the neurone is stimulated, the membrane suddenly changes, electrically charged particles of sodium rush into the cell and potassium rushes out of the cell, causing an electrical current to pass along a section of the neurone. This is called an impulse *action potential* and each one lasts for only a fraction of a second. The process is called conduction (see Figure 1.5).

Some neurones have an insulating wrapping, called *myelin*, which conducts impulses quickly, as the impulse jumps from one break in the myelin, called a *node*, to another. Myelinated nerve fibres can be thought of as fast trains in our analogy, and unmyelinated fibres can be thought of as slow trains that 'stop at all stations'. For example, Louise (see case study in the section on How to Use this Book), has multiple sclerosis, which is caused by problems of myelinated nerve conduction in the sensory nerves and the motor nerves supplying voluntary and involuntary muscle. The myelin has become damaged and patchy and the signals are not conducted smoothly and effectively. This gives rise to different symptoms according to which nerves are affected. The disease will often involve visual disturbances, balance and gait problems, co-ordination of hand and limb movements, an underactive bowel and either overactive or underactive bladder. It is often accompanied by sensation disturbances such as hypersensitivity and by depressed mood.

For Louise, the conduction disturbance has also led to a burning sensation in her legs, weakness in her left leg, reduced perineal sensation and disturbed bladder function, since the myelin damage has affected these nerve pathways the most. Table 1.1 summarises the symptoms.

Other problems such as diabetes or degeneration, which arise from other toxic causes, can also damage myelin. These are generally known as *neuropathies*. Another term that may be used is the ending '-itis' as in *neuritis*, which literally means inflammation or infection of a neurone or neurones. One further term used is *neuralgia* which is an overall term to describe severe pain along the course of a nerve that may be caused by virus, trauma, tumour pressure or inflammation. It is similar to the term *neuropathic pain*, which Chapter 3 discusses in more depth.

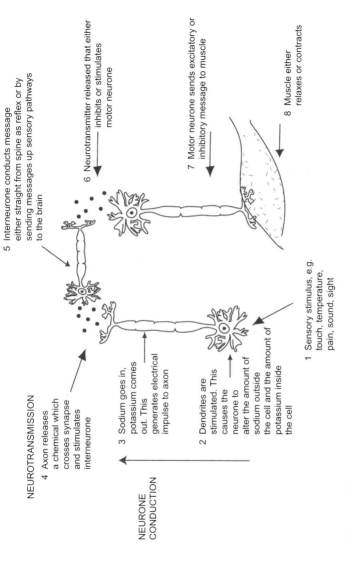

5 Interneurone conducts message either straight from spine as reflex or by sending messages up sensory pathways to the brain

6 Neurotransmitter released that either inhibits or stimulates motor neurone

7 Motor neurone sends excitatory or inhibitory message to muscle

8 Muscle either relaxes or contracts

NEUROTRANSMISSION

4 Axon releases a chemical which crosses synapse and stimulates interneurone

3 Sodium goes in, potassium comes out. This generates electrical impulse to axon

2 Dendrites are stimulated. This causes the neurone to alter the amount of sodium outside the cell and the amount of potassium inside the cell

1 Sensory stimulus, e.g. touch, temperature, pain, sound, sight

NEURONE CONDUCTION

Figure 1.5 Diagram to show nerve conduction and transmission.

Table 1.1 Altered sensation motor ability and cognition.

	Cause	Sensation	Motor ability	Perception and cognition
Motor neurone disease	Degeneration of motor nerves themselves	Not usually affected	May affect limbs, breathing and swallowing	Intelligence and awareness unaffected
Parkinson's disease	Underproduction of neurotransmitter dopamine	Not affected initially	Tremor, rigidity, shuffling walk	Slowed thought processes and dementia may develop in the later stages
Multiple sclerosis	Degeneration of the protective sheath of myelin	Tactile numbness, pins and needles, hypersensitivity	Muscle weakness, fatigue, poor co-ordination	Visual disturbance, slowed thought processes

Transmission of message across a synapse

Another group of diseases which produce neurological symptoms arise from neurotransmitter disturbances. After the action potential has reached the end of the axon, a chemical called a *neurotransmitter* is released. The transmitter crosses the gap between the two neurones. Receptors on the second neurone are then stimulated by the neurotransmitter. In turn, they stimulate the dendrites of the second neurone, which generates an impulse along its length. The communication between nerve cells is called *neurotransmission* (see Figure 1.5).

The amount of neurotransmitter released depends partly on the frequency of the impulses. The more frequent the impulses or messages in the first neurone, the greater the amount of neurotransmitter released at the axon end. The contact point or gap between neurones is called a *synapse*, and different neurons release different transmitters across synapses, which may be inhibitory or excitatory. The synapse is *excitatory* when the neurotransmitter stimulates the second neurone to fire. Synapses are inhibitory when the neurotransmitter restrains the second (postsynaptic) neurone from firing. The first neurone is called *presynaptic* and the second neurone is called *postsynaptic*.

As an example, touching a very hot object usually triggers a reflex withdrawal of the hand to stop the pain. This is because the sensation causes an *excitatory* response. However, if by withdrawing your hand you will be dropping a very expensive piece of ovenware, your brain can send inhibitory signals to block the action. Whether we withdraw our hand or 'hang on' depends on which is stronger the excitatory input – from our sensation, or the inhibitory input from our brain. This complex decision making can be faulty when the part of the brain that evaluates sensation and reasoned action is damaged. Two neurological diseases caused by neurotransmitter disturbance are Parkinson's disease and epilepsy or seizures.

Fred, who has Parkinson's disease (see case study in the section on How to Use this Book), is experiencing 'on' and 'off' periods caused by alterations in the level of the neurotransmitter dopamine. This neurotransmitter is released from motor nerves in the lower part of the brain which initiate voluntary movements through the motor pathways that stimulate activities such as getting up, walking and writing. When the levels are very low there is not enough to stimulate an action potential in a motor neurone, and Fred 'freezes' or has an 'off' period. Table 1.1 summarises these symptoms.

Harry (see case study), who has some brain damage following his sub-arachnoid haemorrhage, may be experiencing seizure activity, which is common after brain injury. His repetitive movements, plucking at sheets and rearranging his sheets may be partial seizure activity. This is abnormal electrical activity in the brain, during which he experiences a change in consciousness, altered motor control and abnormal sensory perceptions. It is included under this section of neurotransmission as anticonvulsant medication often succeeds by modifying neurotransmitter activity.

Other causes of neuronal disturbance

Dehydration and altered levels of the electrolytes in the blood may also cause acute and generalised confusion, because the action potentials and the clear conduction of signals relies on water, sodium and potassium levels that are within normal range. Sodium and potassium imbalance in the body can cause serious disturbances in nerve conduction and transmission. Electrolyte disturbance may be a possible contributory factor in the wandering, confusion and general mood of patients similar to Harry, Mark, Ella or Miriam (see case studies). Patients who are delirious (sometimes described as 'confused') have disturbed levels of consciousness, problems with attention, thinking, perception, emotion, memory, hallucination, and the sleep–wake cycle, and may hallucinate. An abrupt onset of some of these symptoms may indicate delirium. Correcting the electrolyte and hydration problem can often reverse the condition or considerably improve mental functioning.

ORGANISATION AND INTEGRATION OF NEURONES INTO TRACTS, PATHWAYS AND GANGLIA

A *tract* is a bundle of nerve fibres in the brain and spinal cord that are arranged in pathways. *Motor pathways* conduct motor impulses from motor centres in the brain through upper motor neurones and connect through the lower motor neurones to the peripheral system. Impulses along these stimulate a response in muscles or glands. The upper motor neurones have the effect of inhibiting or damping down muscle tone.

Joyce (see case study in the section on How to Use this Book) has suffered a brain injury that has caused painful *spasticity* in her lower limb muscles. This has happened because the spinal reflex that increases muscle tone is no longer inhibited by messages from the upper motor neurones. On the other hand, Irene (see case study) is suffering from disease of the lower motor neurones, which has caused the muscles of her leg to become weak. This has also affected the motor neurones supplying her lungs, causing her to have a reduced breathing efficiency. So both Joyce and Irene have damage to the motor neurones themselves whereas Fred's problems are caused by absent or low levels of the neurotransmitter dopamine, which prevents the motor pathway from being stimulated enough to produce effective muscle contraction and movement.

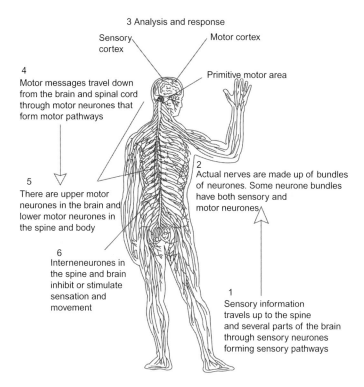

3 Analysis and response

Sensory cortex

Motor cortex

Primitive motor area

4
Motor messages travel down from the brain and spinal cord through motor neurones that form motor pathways

2
Actual nerves are made up of bundles of neurones. Some neurone bundles have both sensory and motor neurones

5
There are upper motor neurones in the brain and lower motor neurones in the spine and body

6
Interneurones in the spine and brain inhibit or stimulate sensation and movement

1
Sensory information travels up to the spine and several parts of the brain through sensory neurones forming sensory pathways

Figure. 1.6 Direction of sensory and motor nerve messages and the role of interneurones.

Sensory pathways conduct sensory (afferent) nerve impulses from various kinds of sensory receptors from the peripheral system to the spinal cord and brain (see Figure 1.6). Louise is suffering from pins and needles, reduced sensitivity or hypersensitivity because the myelin round the nerves in this pathway is affected by her multiple sclerosis.

In addition to these main pathways and central processing in the brain, some neurones are organised in *ganglia* and *nuclei*. These are like very primitive 'mini-brains' or mini sorting stations that can deal with reflexes and primitive responses.

A *ganglion* is a cluster of nerve tissue, usually *outside* the brain and spinal cord. The main types of ganglia are those that contain the cell bodies of sensory neurones that form a chain outside the vertebral column from the neck to the coccyx. These are important in automatic responses such as shivering or some reflexes such as blinking.

With someone like Anwah (see case study in the section on How to Use this Book), it would be very difficult to estimate how she experiences sensation, since the extent of her brain damage seems to indicate that perceptual and cognitive areas of her brain have been heavily affected. Her peripheral sensory receptors and pathways may be intact, but the sensory processing area in the brain is damaged. Consequently, she may have a reflex response to stimulation but not be processing and analysing the sensation in the cortex of her brain.

A *nucleus* is a cluster of neuron cell bodies (grey matter) *inside* the brain or spinal cord that is isolated from the rest of the 'grey matter' by the 'white matter'. The nuclei that are buried in white matter usually have a specific function.

Circuits of sensory, motor, perceptual and cognitive processing

To help integrate incoming information and to co-ordinate responses, the nerve pathways, ganglia, nuclei, interneurones, cell bodies (grey matter), axons and dendrites (white matter) are arranged in circuits or *neuronal pools*. These circuits arrange synapses and neurones in groups called neuronal pools and two main circuit systems that support serial processing and parallel processing as described in Box 1.1. Any patient with a condition that affects this processing capacity, such as stroke, trauma, acquired injury or dementia, is very susceptible to sensory overload that sometimes manifests as agitation or even aggression.

FUNCTIONAL AREAS OF THE BRAIN

The functional areas of the brain are in essence nuclei that are grouped together because they have a specific function, yet are linked by serial and parallel processing circuits. Figures 1.2 (see earlier) and 1.7 show the names of these different regions of grey matter and their main function.

Box 1.1 Types of sensory, motor and cognitive processing

- *Serial processing* occurs where an impulse travels along a single pathway to a specific destination. Reflexes are a good example of this. A *reflex* is an automatic response to a sensory stimulus. Reflexes are specific and predictable, and they can often be protective and help maintain homeostasis. Reflexes are tested in comprehensive medical neurological assessment. Nurses also assess some reflexes when assessing a person's level of consciousness or swallowing ability.
- *Parallel processing* occurs when an impulse travels along several different pathways to be processed and integrated in different parts of the nervous system. Many of the neurones involved will have many branches to their dendrites and axons to allow for many simultaneous synapses. For example, the sensation of pain diverges to several other pathways leading to different parts of the brain for evaluation. This type of processing occurs in complex mental functions. Nursing assessment of perceptual and cognitive factors such as orientation to time, place and person involves some aspects of parallel processing activity.

Lobes of the brain

The higher brain is called the *cortex* and is made up of numerous cell bodies, giving it a grey appearance. This layer of grey cells has areas of specific function, called *lobes* (see Figure 1.7). The cortex is where activities such as reasoning and problem solving take place, and we might refer colloquially to someone we deem clever as 'not being short of old grey matter'. As shown in Figure 1.2, the midbrain contains the thalamus and hypothalamus, areas where we register feeling and mood as well as where appetite and body temperature are regulated.

Mark (see case study in the section on How to Use this Book) may have some damage to this area, resulting in disturbed regulation of eating and no feeling of satiety. He may also have damage to the frontal lobes. This may result in behavioural

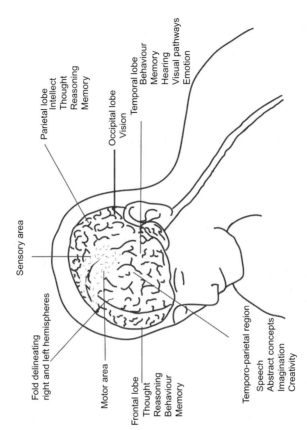

Figure 1.7 Functions of the lobes of the cortex of the brain.

Parietal lobe
Intellect
Thought
Reasoning
Memory

Occipital lobe
Vision

Temporal lobe
Behaviour
Memory
Hearing
Visual pathways
Emotion

Sensory area

Fold delineating
right and left hemispheres

Motor area

Frontal lobe
Thought
Reasoning
Behaviour
Memory

Temporo-parietal region
Speech
Abstract concepts
Imagination
Creativity

problems, which are common after brain injury, because very primitive aggressive responses in these areas are no longer inhibited by the calming influence of the cortex.

Hemispheres of the brain

The lobes are also in hemispheres – right and left – that appear to be mirror images. Functionally, however, one hemisphere is usually dominant. In most people, the left hemisphere is dominant for reading, writing, understanding, speaking and sequencing movements, such as reaching and grasping.

The right hemisphere has a greater capacity to process spatial and visual information, and gives rise to imagination and an appreciation of music. Ella (see case study in the section on How to Use this Book) has suffered a stroke or clot in the left hemisphere of her brain. Because the left side of the brain controls the motor pathways on the right side of the body, she has a motor deficit on the right side of the body. She has a language disturbance because the area of the brain concerned with language is in the left hemisphere, and she has a swallowing problem because the cranial nerves co-ordinating her swallowing are damaged, but she may well be able to sing, hum and enjoy a good imagination.

Protection of the brain

The nervous system is so crucial to our well-being that it has several kinds of protection, including the following:

- The skull and vertebra of the backbone.
- Three layers of tough connective tissue called the *meninges*.
- *Cerebrospinal fluid*, which is a nutritive and protective fluid flowing round the brain and spinal cord through a series of connected chambers, called *ventricles*.
- A circular blood supply called the *Circle of Willis*. These blood vessels form a ring at the base of the brain that form a 'backup' blood supply if one of the arteries is blocked (see Figure 1.8). This can help minimise damage to the brain tissue from a clot or rupture.
- *Arterioles*, which have tight junctions that prevent many substances and pathogens passing through to brain tissue. This

is called the blood–brain barrier. Alcohol and some drugs are able to pass through this barrier, and pathogens can enter if there is damage to it.

- *Neuroglial* cells that surround neuronal tissue and ingest and destroy bacteria and debris.

Neurological impairments can occur when one or more of these protective mechanisms are breached or become diseased and neurones become damaged as shown in Box 1.2. In the case studies, Mark, Joyce and Gary have suffered trauma, Anwah has suffered an infection of the meninges (meningitis), Harry, Miriam and Ella have acquired brain damage through disrup-

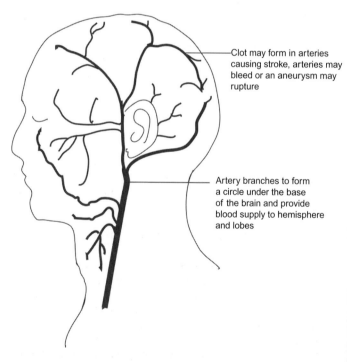

Clot may form in arteries causing stroke, arteries may bleed or an aneurysm may rupture

Artery branches to form a circle under the base of the brain and provide blood supply to hemisphere and lobes

Figure 1.8 Blood vessels supplying the brain.

Box 1.2 Impairment in the defences of the nervous system

- A clot may form in a blood vessel (see Figure 1.8).
- A damaged blood vessel may leak into the brain tissue.
- Blood or pus may contaminate cerebrospinal fluid and be circulated around the nervous system.
- A blockage may develop between the chambers of the ventricles and cause hydrocephalus and raised pressure in the brain.
- An abscess may develop or the meninges may become infected.
- Toxins from drugs can cross over the blood–brain barrier and cause confusion or altered consciousness.
- Disturbances in body chemistry such as uraemia or hypoxia can cause disturbed brain function.
- Tumours may arise in the neuroglial cells.

---

tion to the blood supply to the brain, and Louise has degeneration of the protective myelin around some neurones. Table 1.2 gives examples of the conditions and impairments that may occur.

CONNECTION BETWEEN CENTRAL NERVOUS SYSTEM PERIPHERAL NERVES

The spinal cord is a continuation of primitive brain tissue extending from the base of the skull to the first lumbar vertebra in the lower back. It carries the sensory and motor pathways that connect to the *cranial* and *spinal* nerves that form the peripheral system (see Tables 1.3 and 1.4 and Figure 1.1). Each peripheral nerve has sensory responsibility for a specific segment of skin called a *dermatome* and motor responsibility for a specific muscle.

Table 1.2 Impairments and diseases.

Term	Comments	Causes	Manifestations
Stroke	Sub-arachnoid haemorrhage may also be considered here	Disturbance in the blood supply to the brain either because of a clot or haemorrhage. Lack of oxygen to the portion of nerve tissue the artery supplies gives rise to neurological symptoms	Will depend very much on which artery is affected and how much of the brain it supplies. People may have wide variation in the degree of altered sensation, motor ability, perception and cognition. Very often affects one side of the body only
Dementia	Not a discrete disease but a group of symptoms that demonstrate a decline of mental abilities accompanied by changes in personality and behaviour	Degeneration of the neurone, such as in Alzheimer's disease, multiple clots in the brain arteries, and also non-neurological causes such as nutritional deficiencies, thyroid disease or depression	People who suffer from dementia will also have wide variation in the degree and severity of their impairments. One of the most troublesome of these may be memory
Aphasia	Also called dysphasia, an impairment of the power of expression by speech, writing or signs, or of comprehending spoken or written language, due to injury or disease of the temporo-parietal lobe in right-handed people. Can be confused with *dysarthria*	It can be caused by many neurological conditions and needs to be thoroughly assessed to ascertain capability as well as disability	Difficulty in word finding, saying the wrong but loosely connected word, muddling yes and no. In some types people may invent words
Dysarthria	There may be no involvement of the higher brain, language ability or perception	Weakness of muscles of face and throat. Commonly experienced by people with motor neurone disease or multiple sclerosis, certain kinds of stroke or haemorrhage, brain tumour or congenital problem	Difficulty in forming words, resulting in slurred speech. Lack of intonation, low volume, sometimes nasal
Apraxia	The term used when a person with neurological injury or degeneration shows an inability to perform purposeful movements although no muscular paralysis or sensory disturbance is present	Any traumatic, congenital or acquired brain injury. It is often a problem of planning and sequencing and demonstrates a disturbance of parallel processing	Difficulty in working out how to stand up, reach for a cup and hold it to the mouth, getting dressed

Table 1.3 Cranial nerves and the effects of damage.

Name of cranial nerve	Function	Possible problem
Olfactory (I) (sensory)	Smell	Absence or distortion
Optic (II) (sensory)	Vision	Disturbed visual field, possibly following stroke (hemianopia)
Oculomotor (III) (motor)	Pupil constriction Lens accommodation Eyeball movement	Double vision Pressure from oedema in the brain
Trochlea (IV) (motor)	Downward and inward eye movement	Double vision
Trigeminal (V) (motor and sensory)	Sensation to the face, scalp, teeth, lips, eyeballs, nose and throat lining Proprioception of muscles used for chewing	Decreased facial sensation and motor function may be due to neuralgia, brain injury, motor neurone disease, multiple sclerosis
Abducens (VI) (motor)	Sideways eye movements	Paralysis
Facial (VII) (motor and sensory)	Muscles of the face used in facial expression	Decreased strength and drooping of the face due to brain or cranial nerve damage as in Parkinson's disease, MND, MS or brain injury
Acoustic (VIII) (sensory) Also known as vestibulocochlear	Hearing Balance	Deafness or dizziness
Glossopharyngeal (IX) (motor and sensory)	Proprioception of throat muscles used in swallowing Speech production and sensation in the pharynx Taste Saliva and tear production	Speech 'slurring' (dysarthria) and swallowing problems (dysphagia)
Vagus (X) (motor and sensory)	Sensation from lungs, heart liver, pancreas, stomach, kidneys, intestines and reproductive organs. Regulation of heart rate, airflow, peristalsis, reproductive activities Swallowing Speech	Disturbances of digestive or elimination function Dysarthria or dysphagia as above
Spinal accessory (XI) (motor)	Soft palate movement Head rotation	Reduced strength in neck and shoulders Dysphagia
Hypoglossal (XII) (motor)	Tongue and throat movements in speech and swallowing	Dysarthria Dysphagia

Table 1.4 Spinal nerves.

Spinal nerves	Broad area served
Cervical nerves (8 pairs, C1–C8)	Head, neck and parts of shoulders and arms
Thoracic nerves (12 pairs, T1–T12)	Inner aspect of the arm and most of the trunk
Lumbar nerves (5 pairs, L1–L5)	Pelvis and legs. Spinal cord ends at L2 and branches into cauda equina, the name for where all the other remaining nerves leave the spine
Sacral nerves (5 pairs, S1–S5)	Perineum, buttocks and thighs, foot and ankle
Coccygeal (1 pair)	Coccyx

- The 12 pairs of *cranial nerves* are attached to the brainstem. Some of these nerves are sensory, some are motor and some are mixed. They supply the face, throat and neck. One in particular, the vagus nerve, also supplies the head, chest and organs of the abdomen
- The 31 pairs of *spinal nerves* connect with the spinal cord at different points along the vertebra of the neck, thorax, lumbar and sacral region. They are named according to the vertebra with which they are associated, and are mixed sensory and motor nerves

PERIPHERAL NERVE PROBLEMS (NEUROPATHY)

Neuropathy can often develop from other conditions and diseases such as badly controlled diabetes, excess alcohol intake or environmental toxins and some drugs. One other particular neuropathy worth remembering in a general care setting is *critical-illness neuropathy*. This can develop in up to 50% of patients who have been in a critical care unit for more than two weeks (Rolak 1998). There may be marked weakness of respiratory muscles, sensory loss and weakness.

It is possible that Miriam is experiencing some degree of *peripheral neuropathy*, given the length of time she was in High Dependency, and the possibility that she may have been difficult to wean from a ventilator. Time, good nutrition and hydration and a period of care will usually ensure a good recovery. The most common primary neurological condition causing neuropathy, however, is *Guillain-Barré,* syndrome, which can develop a few weeks after a febrile illness. The main symptoms are usually weakness, which may affect the thoracic muscles and breathing. Recovery after a period of weeks or months, with appropriate care and treatment, is usual.

THE AUTONOMIC NERVES

The main difference between autonomic and other nerves is the kind of tissue that the nerve contacts. The autonomic (involuntary) nerves

- contact glands and internal organs, and
- regulate activities such as the heart rate, sweating, stomach contractions and the size of the pupil of the eye (see Fig 1.3).

By contrast, the somatic (voluntary) nerves

- contact skeletal muscle, and
- regulate voluntary movement.

Classification of autonomic nerves

Autonomic nerves are either *sympathetic* or *parasympathetic*. The sympathetic nerves keep the body in a state of readiness for action whereas the parasympathetic nerves keep the body calm and peaceful. Much autonomic activity is modulated by the ganglia outside the vertebral column. Although activity is often maintained at the spinal level, emotional states of mind or disturbance of brain tissue can affect their functioning. This is the reason why stress and anxiety can produce physiological symptoms such as changes in heart rate and rhythm, breathing rate, disturbances of digestion, menstruation and elimination, and sweating. Damage to the spinal nerves can also manifest as autonomic disturbance. Table 1.5 summarises some potential problems in peripheral nerve and autonomic nerve function.

PERSONALITY, MOOD AND BEHAVIOUR

While human beings are similar in general anatomical design and physiological function, each person is a unique blend of

Table 1.5 Disturbances of the peripheral nervous system.

Condition	Cause	Symptoms	Intervention	Nursing comment
Guillain-Barré syndrome (GBS)	An acute inflammation of the peripheral nerves that may be so severe as to threaten life because of the weakness of the respiratory muscles	The symptoms are usually weakness, loss of reflexes and loss of sensations such as proprioception, pain, hot and cold, touch, pressure and vibration	Mechanical ventilation may be needed until the inflammation has subsided and the function returns	From a nursing point of view the impaired sensation and motor loss put these patients at very high risk of developing pressure sores and of being unable to protect themselves in other ways. For example, the cough reflex or swallowing reflex may be impaired. Abrupt and dangerous fluctuations in blood pressure regulation that need to be monitored
Autonomic dysreflexia	Damage in spinal nerves T6 to T8. Autonomic dysreflexia can arise if bladder and bowel elimination are not properly managed. The reflex that bladder or bowel fullness generates is disordered and an uncontrolled disturbance of autonomic function develops that dangerously deranges homeostasis	Sudden rise in blood pressure Slowing pulse Sweating Severe headache Gooseflesh	Reduce blood pressure Drain urinary bladder safely by catheterisation Remove other potential triggers Educate patient about complications	Vulnerable patient should have clear bowel and bladder management programmes
Disturbances that may be associated with other neurological conditions, e.g. Parkinson's disease, multiple sclerosis, epilepsy	Underactivity or overactivity of nerves caused by neurotransmitter imbalance, damage to myelin sheath or degeneration of neurone	Postural hypotension, loss of sweating or excessive sweating, dry mouth and eyes, disordered micturition and elimination, impotence or other genito-urinary problems	Medication to control symptoms Care plan to minimise safety risk, maximise independence and provide practical comfort management	Risk of falls, hydration problems, skin reactions. Loss of continence, pressure sore risk, altered body image, low self-esteem

genetic, psychological and cultural, environmental and socio-political influences. These are expressed through personality, mood and behaviour. In anatomical terms, it is thought that the midbrain and the frontal lobe have an important role in learning appropriate and inappropriate behaviours. Damage to the frontal lobe of the brain can result in an apathetic mood and a lack of initiative arising from spontaneous motivation.

Miriam, for example, may be suffering apathy from the effects of frontal lobe damage, particularly if the haemorrhage she suffered supplied this area. On the other hand, cursing, uttering obscenities, tactlessness and lack of self-control can also indicate that there is damage to the frontal lobes. The brain damage that Harry has suffered may be frontal and manifesting as his inappropriate behaviour towards the nurses and his restlessness.

People who have dementia, which can be diffuse throughout the brain, may experience different symptoms as the disease progresses: levels of attention and concentration drop and short-term memory is poor. They may become fatuous, overemotional or indifferent. These behaviours are governed by their immediate needs rather than by normal social interactions.

Mood and personality are very often disturbed in neurological illness for obvious psychological reason as well as for neurological ones. If you look through all the case studies once more, you will see that nearly all the patients are manifesting some kind of disturbance. Skill lies in differentiating between physiological and psychological causes and the interactions between the two.

SUMMARY
❏ Neurones are the basic structure of the nervous system and they communicate sensory and motor messages by conduction and transmission.
❏ Successful conduction of a message along its length needs an intact neurone, balanced levels of sodium and potassium and a good blood supply.
❏ Successful transmission of a message across a synapse from one neurone to another needs intact axons and dendrites, an adequate supply of either excitatory or inhibitory neurotransmitter, and a healthy blood supply.

❏ Neurones are organised in bundles that form sensory or motor pathways that are capable of simple reflexes at the spinal level or connected by a complex of ganglia and interneurones that support parallel processing. This accounts for higher-level functions such as memory, cognition, reasoning, language, personality and our individuality.

❏ Neurological impairment occurs after trauma, after degeneration of specific neurones such as in motor neurone disease, degeneration or inflammation of the myelin protecting neurones as in multiple sclerosis or Guillain-Barré syndrome. It may also occur after disturbance of the blood supply to brain tissue as in stroke or sub-arachnoid haemorrhage or after imbalance in the amount of neurotransmitter being released as in Parkinson's disease or epilepsy.

❏ The autonomic nerves maintain basic body functions such as heart rate, blood pressure, peristalsis, digestion, elimination, body temperature control and hormonal activity. They work without conscious control but can be affected by mood and emotional state and in some cases, such as defecation, are supplied with voluntary muscle through which people learn voluntary control.

❏ Most neurological impairments can be described under the terms altered sensation, altered motor ability, altered perception or altered cognition.

❏ Personality, mood and behaviour can be affected by neurological impairments as either a direct effect of anatomical and physiological dysfunction or a valid psychological response to health breakdown, or a combination of both.

REFERENCE

Rolak, L. A. (1998) *Neurology Secrets*, 2nd edn. Hanley & Belfus, Philadelphia.

BIBLIOGRAPHY

Adams, R. D. and Victor, M. (1994) *Principles of Neurology Companion Handbook*, 5th edn. McGraw-Hill, New York.

Axford, J. and O'Callaghan, C. (2004) *Medicine*, 2nd edn. Blackwell, Oxford.

Bastian, G. F. (1993) *An Illustrated Review of the Nervous System*. HarperCollins College Publishers, New York.

Hickey, J. (1997) *The Clinical Practice of Neurological and Neurosurgical Nursing*, 4th edn. Lippincott, Philadelphia.

Lasserson, D., Gabriel, C. and Sharrack, B. (1998) *Nervous System and Special Senses*. Mosby, London.

Liebman, M. (1979) *Neuroanatomy Made Easy and Understandable*. University Park Press, Baltimore.

Marieb, E. (1992) *Human Anatomy and Physiology*, 2nd edn. Benjamin Cummings, California.

Rolak, L. A. (1998) *Neurology Secrets*, 2nd edn. Hanley & Belfus, Philadelphia.

Rutishauser, S. (1994) *Physiology and Anatomy: A Basis for Nursing and Healthcare*. Churchill Livingstone, Edinburgh.

Wilson, K. J. W. (1987) *Ross and Wilson Anatomy and Physiology in Health and Illness*, 6th edn. Churchill Livingstone, Edinburgh.

2 | Nursing Assessment

INTRODUCTION

This chapter focuses on the techniques nurses use to assess baseline neurological function and how to identify physical changes or impairments that may cause actual or potential problems in the activities of living. Nursing assessment is a cyclical activity that collects information from a patient, reviews it and then uses it both to identify any difficulties the person has in the activities of living and to prioritise those problems. This includes assessing level of consciousness, sensation, motor ability, balance and co-ordination, perceptual and cognitive function and peripheral nerve function. The techniques suggested include using structured observation tools such as the Glasgow Coma Scale, collecting data that can be observed and measured, and using unstructured means such as interview, conversation and interpersonal interaction to collect subjective information. A high blood pressure, for example, is objective data, whereas having a dreadful headache is an example of subjective data. This baseline neurological assessment is used to detect improvement or deterioration and the implications for all the activities of living.

Although the focus here is primarily on nursing assessment, interprofessional working is an important part of the overall care planning. Doctors carry out a structured neurological physical assessment and initiate laboratory tests and specialist neurological investigations that provide further objective data. Physiotherapists assess movement, gait, balance and muscle power. Occupational therapists assess perceptual and cognitive function and other aspects of physical functioning that may affect self-care ability. Speech and language therapists assess ability to communicate and the swallowing function. The assessments carried out by this team can be useful sources of information for nurses. Some wards and units use interdisciplinary care pathways and collaborative notes. These help integrate assessment by different members of the team in the care planning process (Kirrane 2000). Nurses, however, are in the unique position of being able to assess and reassess patients throughout the 24 hours, through all the activities of living and through the development of a therapeutic relationship with them (Hickey 1997; Stewart-Amidei and Kunkel 2001). A growing familiarity with a patient can help nurses assess subtle changes in physical or psychological well-being that could be early indicators of a worsening condition or of complications or secondary problems developing.

LEARNING OUTCOMES

❏ Outline the key techniques used in a nursing assessment of a patient's level of consciousness, orientation and cognition, motor function, sensory function, balance and co-ordination.
❏ Describe how to correctly assess and interpret changes in observed data such as temperature, pulse, respiration rate, blood pressure and pulse oximetry that may indicate developing problems.
❏ Appreciate the role of an interdisciplinary co-operation in assessment, and the role of the nurse within that team.
❏ Outline the main purpose of common neurological tests and investigations.

INITIAL ASSESSMENT

The quality of the initial assessment is crucial since it is used as the basis of comparison over time to establish whether there is improvement, stabilisation or deterioration. In carrying out an assessment, a nurse needs to

- decide what to assess;
- use the proper technique for assessment;
- use an appropriate method of documentation;
- know how to interpret the findings;
- know what action to take (Lehman *et al.* 2003).

All of the above involve not only well-developed reasoning power and clinical decision making, but also good observational, interpersonal and practical skills (Hickey 1997). Sources that contribute to a thorough assessment include:

- a detailed discussion with the patient themselves when possible covering the points mentioned in Box 2.1;
- previous nursing records;
- medical records and documentation of other members of the health care team;
- structured neurological and generalised assessment sheets;
- diagnostic test results;
- family and friends.

Synthesis of these sources should ensure that the assessment is thorough and based on objective and subjective, structured and unstructured data.

GENERAL OBSERVATIONS

Routine observations of pulse, respiration rate, blood pressure and temperature may indicate disturbances of the autonomic system that are neurologically significant. The following abnormalities could indicate deterioration in the patient's condition.

Box 2.1 Broad areas to assess

- Past or present problems with level of consciousness, motor function, sensation, memory, thought processes, speech, intellectual function, fainting, dizziness, headache, seizures or head injury.
- Social history including education, employment, alcohol consumption and family history of neurological disorders.
- Sleep disturbances, insomnia, wandering behaviour, daytime sleepiness or sleep apnoea.
- Personality changes, confusion, lethargy, depression, mood swings or aggressiveness.
- Bowel or bladder disturbance and continence.
- Medications, tranquillisers, sedatives or anticonvulsants.
- Allergies.
- Vital signs.

Pulse

A slowing pulse and a widening pulse pressure (the difference between the systolic and the diastolic pressure) could indicate an increasing pressure inside the skull (intracranial pressure) and potentially life-threatening deterioration (Edwards 2001). A rapid pulse may indicate fluctuations in intracranial pressure, and cardiac arrhythmias may occur in patients with a sub-arachnoid haemorrhage or severe head injury (Hickey 1997).

Respiration

The rate, depth and rhythm of breathing can indicate whether the vital functions of the brain stem are compromised. Also, secretions may cause noisy breathing and render the person vulnerable to aspiration, a risk associated with a variety of neurological conditions.

Pulse oximetry

Normal values lie between 95% and 100%, and a falling pattern can alert practitioners to a developing oxygenation problem. An oxygen saturation level of less than 90% is usually a cause for concern, even though there may not be any cyanosis. Pulse oximetry, however, does not provide information about the carbon dioxide levels and may fail to detect the acidosis that develops from retained carbon dioxide. It may help Irene (see case study in the section on How to Use this Book) if overnight pulse oximetry is carried out. This can then give an oxygen saturation pattern that can be sent to the laboratory for analysis, and guide treatment options.

Blood pressure

A rising blood pressure together with a slowing pulse can indicate *rising intracranial pressure* (Shah 1999; Woodrow 2000) in brain injured patients or any condition which has the potential to increase the pressure inside the skull mechanically or chemically. *Raised intracranial pressure* is very serious and can develop very quickly. Harry (see case study), during his period of excessive sleepiness, may be experiencing raised intracranial pressure due to his earlier haemorrhage; or if his blood pressure is raised and his pulse slow, and this is unusual for him, he may be having further cerebral bleeding.

Other disturbances of autonomic function, such as overstimulation or understimulation of the sympathetic nerves of the thalamus and spine, may cause blood pressure disturbances and cardiac arrhythmias (Hickey 1997).

Mark (see case study) has an unsteady and uneven gait and lolls to one side while sitting. There could be several reasons such as hemiplegia, brain stem damage, damage to acoustic nerve or ear drum, dizziness, or loss of proprioception. However, if temperature, pulse and respiration (TPR) and blood pressure (BP) readings are abnormal, this may indicate that the autonomic system is struggling to maintain homeostasis. The blood pressure may drop on standing or when exerting, or there may be cardiac arrhythmias, which are contributing to unsteadiness and dizziness. Nurses could initiate a lying and standing blood pressure recording, and a pulse and apex recording and an ECG may be ordered. If there are abnormalities, these can be corrected with medication thereby preventing potential cardiac problems from developing.

Ella (see case study) will need her BP, pulse, oxygen saturations and blood glucose levels monitored every four hours during the early days after her stroke. If they show no abnormalities they will be checked either once or twice daily after one week. Often, a patient's blood pressure will be higher post stroke as an autonomic response to maintain cerebral perfusion. Ella's pulse must be observed for regularity and strength, since the blood clot causing the stroke could have originated in the heart. Ella's oxygen saturations and respirations are the most sensitive indicators for any worsening of her condition.

Temperature

A raised temperature may indicate infection, but in neurological patients with possible brain involvement it may indicate a problem with the hypothalamus, (situated in the midbrain) because it has a role in regulating body temperature (Hickey 1997). For example, Ella's temperature should be kept below 37°C and her blood sugar maintained within normal limits. This will help to maintain a stable environment within her body, which will prevent further damage and minimise the neurological impact of the stroke.

RAISED INTRACRANIAL PRESSURE

Pressure inside the brain, caused by traumatic brain injury, cerebral bleed or stroke, can develop rapidly and is dangerous because of the downward pressure on the centres controlling breathing and heart rate, and blood pressure. Rising intracranial pressure is a medical emergency and needs to be assessed and managed by a specialist emergency or neuroscience practitioner. Close attention to the vital signs and assessment of the level of consciousness using the Glasgow Coma Scale can pick up the signs that the pressure is rising and prompt early intervention. For example, early intubation and ventilation can reduce the pressure in the skull and prevent secondary injury from serious impairment of blood flow to the brain tissue which was initially unaffected by the injury or insult (Hickey 1997).

ASSESSING THE LEVEL OF CONSCIOUSNESS

Alertness depends on the state of the *reticular activating system (RAS)* which can be affected by a range of different conditions as shown in Box 2.2. The RAS is a network of brain tissue extending from the centre core of the brain stem to all parts of the cerebral cortex. The system is important in

• producing sleep states and awakening mechanisms;
• maintaining arousal and awareness;
• modulation of sensory information, pain and respiration;
• the integration of autonomic functions.

All patients in the case studies have the potential for altered level of consciousness, either in the early stages of their injury, because of seizure activity following injury, or because of reduced blood flow and oxygen levels in the brain. However, the most serious developments in intracranial pressure usually occur in the first few hours after injury, toxicity or hypoxaemia. Damage to the system from trauma, haemorrhage or disordered metabolism can bring about a lowering of the level of consciousness and potentially serious consequences. The National Institute for Clinical Excellence has produced guidelines and a

---

Box 2.2 Possible causes of altered level of consciousness

- Infarctions, tumours, abscesses or trauma – all of which may lead to oedema and raised intracranial pressure.
- Aneurysms, haemorrhages.
- Lack of energy substrates – oxygen, low blood sugar, vitamin deficiency.
- Toxic effects of drugs, particularly opiates, steroids, sedatives.
- Metabolic toxicity such as uraemia in kidney disease, liver disease and electrolyte disturbance.

Commonest causes

- Hypoxia
- Hypoglycaemia
- Sedative drug overdose

---

series of algorithms to ensure that people who have suffered traumatic brain injury receive appropriate referral and timely interventions to protect the brain from secondary damage (NICE 2002).

Using the Glasgow Coma Scale

The most common tool nurses use to estimate level of consciousness is the Glasgow Coma Scale (GCS). The GCS was developed by Teasdale and Jennet (1974) to standardise observations for the objective assessment of the level of consciousness. The simple numerical scale allocates a value to a patient's best responses to stimuli that involve eye opening, motor response and verbal responses (Box 2.3). The scores are recorded on an observation chart which usually also includes other neurological observations. The lowest possible score is 3, even in patients who are ventilated, sedated and paralysed, as well as in those in very deep coma from pathological processes.

- Patients with a GCS of 13 at any time since traumatic injury or patients with a GCS of 13 or 14 two hours after injury need to be considered, along with other criteria, for CT scan (NICE 2002).

- The observations need to be made frequently, as there may be delayed onset of altered level of consciousness and deterioration may be rapid.
- The scale has been shown to be a useful and reliable practical tool (Juarez and Lyons 1995), but less accurate at the intermediate level of consciousness, of below 12, with inexperienced users (Rowley and Fielding 1991). For this reason, all members of staff need to assess the patient in the same way to ensure reliability (Edwards 2001). In addition, Fairley and Cosgrove (1999) suggest that a local clinical guideline can be developed to standardise the way the GCS is carried out.

Box 2.3 Glasgow Coma Scale

Stimuli response	**Response score**
Eye opening	
Never	1
To pain	2
To verbal stimuli	3
Spontaneously	4
Best verbal response	
No response	1
Incomprehensible sounds	2
Inappropriate word making little sense	3
Converses but confused	4
Orientated to time, place and person	5
Best motor response	
No response to pain	1
Extends all limbs to pain	2
Flexes elbows and wrists, extends legs to pain	3
Withdraws from painful stimulus	4
Localises to source of pain and attempts to remove it	5
Obeys simple verbal command	6

Eye opening

The eye opening response assesses arousal and reactivity. The score may be biased if the person is deaf or has swollen eyes. If the eyes cannot open because of swelling, the nurse should record a C on the recording chart. There may also be weakness of the eyelids because of damage to the oculomotor nerve or other neurological condition such as myasthenia gravis.

There is a range of different techniques to elicit an eye opening response to pain. Frawley (1990) suggests that peripheral nerve stimulation should be used. Shah (1999) asserts that applying pressure to the nail bed is extremely painful and that applying pressure to the side of the finger is sufficient to elicit a response. In addition, Edwards (2001) suggests that nurses may be able to assess eye opening when carrying out care that may itself be painful or irritating, without the need to administer extra pain on a frequent basis.

Verbal response

This explores cognitive function of the higher brain and the patient's states of awareness of their surroundings, time and place. It assesses understanding of what has been said and the ability to express thoughts in words (Jevon and Ewens 2002).

The nurse should ask the patient simple questions, avoiding ones that require just a yes/no answer.

- Time – What day/date/month/season/time is it?
- Place – Where are you now? What is the name of the hospital/town/city? Where do you live?
- Person – What is your name? What is your wife's/partner's name? What job does this person (pointing to nurse/doctor) do? Who is this person (pointing to wife/partner/other person well known to the patient)?

The presence of aphasia may distort the GCS score (see Table 2.1), as would deafness or the presence of a tracheostomy tube. If dysphasia is present, D should be recorded; T should be recorded if a tracheostomy tube is present (Jevon and Ewens 2002).

Table 2.1 Aphasic responses.

	Orientated	Confused	Expressively dysphasic	Receptively dysphasic
What day of the week is it?	Gives correct day	Gives incorrect day	Says 'yes yes yes'	Sticks tongue out
What is the date?	Gives correct date	Gives an incorrect, even outlandish, date	Says 'no no no'	Smiles and points
What is the month?	Gives correct month	Gives incorrect month	Nods and says 'mmmm'	Lifts arms in the air
What is the year?	Gives correct year	Gives incorrect year	Shakes head and waves you away	Closes eyes and appears to go to sleep
Where are you now?	Gives correct response	'I'm at home. What are you doing here?'	Smiles and says 'no, no yes'	Smiles and says 'Do you want a cup of tea?'

Motor response

It is important to remember to record the best motor response (Jevon and Ewens 2002). The most commonly used rating is out of 6, which contains a score linked to withdrawal from pain. Some areas that use an earlier version omit this category.

- The nurse asks the patient to hold up their right arm/thumb. If the patient does not respond to this verbal request, a motor response to pain is assessed.
- A response to pain should elicit cerebral function rather than a spinal nerve reflex and be the least needed. Edwards (2001) suggests that the *trapezium squeeze* is most appropriate, where the muscle at the angle between the neck and shoulders is squeezed using thumb and two fingers. *Supraorbital pressure*, where a finger is run over the bone above the eye, is unsuitable for patients with a brain injury. The *sternal rub*, where the knuckles are rubbed over the sternum, can cause bruising and should not be used. Application of pressure to the nail bed can be traumatic and may only elicit a spinal reflex. If the patient does not respond after 30 seconds, the painful stimulus should stop (Lower 1992). Localising to pain and reaching towards it shows more awareness than flexion to pain (*decorticate posture*), which shows more awareness than extension to pain (*decerebrate posture*).

Further points

- The individual GCS scores are important and can indicate significant changes, particularly the eye opening response, since this can indicate increasing pressure on the lower brain.
- The numerical score needs to be supplemented by observation of the vital signs, assessment of pupil response and limb power. The findings from this may be integrated on a neurological observation chart to facilitate interpretation.
- There is no protocol for the frequency of observations (Edwards 2001). Clinical judgement determines the frequency, with hourly observation being the minimal to detect signs of deterioration, although every 15 minutes is common in an unstable patient.

ADDITIONAL NEUROLOGICAL ASSESSMENT

The GCS is supplemented by observation of blood pressure, respiration rate, pulse rate, temperature, and an estimation of *pupil size and reactivity* and *limb movement and power*. The estimate of pupil size and reaction can detect if there are serious pressure problems in the brain, and an assessment of the power of the limbs can identify motor nerve impairment. The interpretation of pupil responses and appearance takes practice, and inter-rater reliability always needs to be evaluated. Any changes can be very significant and must be attributable to change in the patient rather than a change of observer. The size of the pupils is estimated using a small torch and comparing the pupil with the scale printed on the neurological observation chart before and after the light source. The important features to assess are the size, equality, shape and reactivity to light using a pen torch. The findings of one pupil are always compared with the findings in the other pupil and the differences, if any, between the two are noted. The procedure should go through the following steps:

- Watch the person and see if they open their eyes spontaneously.
- Introduce yourself and ask the person to open their eyes, explaining that you need to assess their pupils using a light.
- If the eyelids do not open to speech, explain that you are going to raise the eyelids and shine a light into their eyes to assess the pupils and that this will not hurt.
- Raise the eyelids and hold open to prevent the blink reflex.
- Estimate the size of the pupil.
- Bring the lit torch towards the eye from the right side of the eye for the right eye and the left side of the eye for the left eye. This overcomes the immediate accommodation response in which the pupils constrict as the eyes converge on a near object.
- Look at the pupils. Are they equal in size? Are they regular in outline? Are there any holes in the iris or foreign bodies?
- Shine the light in one eye.
- Look at the reaction of that eye (this is called the direct reflex), and then repeat and look at the reaction in the eye in which you are not shining the light. This is called the consensual reflex.

- The person should be looking into the distance rather than at the light if possible.
- Repeat for the other eye.

Recording the findings

Normally the pupils are equal in size (about 2–6 mm), and two methods are used to record pupil size. The millimetre scale offers a diagrammatic gauge, usually illustrated on the recording sheet, which shows black circles ranging from 2 mm to 9 mm. The pupil size for each eye should be entered on the recording chart. A reaction time should also be recorded using B for brisk and S for sluggish or N for no reaction. In some areas, verbal descriptors may be used instead, such as pinpoint, small, mid-sized, large or dilated. If one pupil is fixed, dilated and unreactive to light, this can indicate seriously raised intracranial pressure, haematoma or herniation of the brain downwards. If both pupils are fixed and dilated, it indicates severe midbrain damage, cardiopulmonary arrest or poisoning. Mid-sized pupils also indicate midbrain involvement, while pinpoint pupils may be the result of lesions in the pons or the effect of opiates. In the latter case, however, the pupils would respond to the light.

CRANIAL NERVE ASSESSMENT

Nurses in a general care setting do not usually carry out structured cranial nerve examination. The aspects of cranial nerve function relevant to a nursing assessment, such as difficulty in swallowing or communicating verbally, are included in the later chapters.

ASSESSING MUSCLE AND LIMB POWER

An assessment of muscle and limb power can help to detect weakness on one side (hemiparesis), gives an overall picture of motor nerve function and informs risk assessment in relation to patient safety.

- Inspect the muscles of limbs for wasting, comparing right with left. Spastic muscles will stand out visibly, feel abnormally hard and resist if stretched.

- Ask the person to close their eyes and hold their arms out in front, palms up and fingers splayed for 20–30 seconds. This may show tremor or weakness, indicated by one arm drifting away.
- Test handgrips for power and equality by asking the patient to squeeze your index and middle finger as hard as possible. A normal grip strength would mean that it is difficult to remove the fingers from the grip.
- Is the person able to raise a leg in the air while lying down, or to rise from lying to standing. These movements all require sufficient strength to overcome gravity.
- Can the person move the limbs against mild, moderate and strong resistance? Ask them to push the limb against your hand and vary the resistance.
- A medical examination involves a thorough assessment of all upper and lower limb muscle groups and should have been recorded in the medical notes. A rating scale for limb power, as devised by the Medical Research Council (see Box 2.4) may be used and recorded on the neurological observation chart for each limb.

ASSESSING REFLEXES

Assessment of reflexes is usually carried out by a doctor, and the absence, slowed response or abnormal responses of direction or briskness indicates disease or damage at some point in the pathway.

Box 2.4 The MRC scale for muscle power

Grade	Response
0	No movement
1	Flicker of muscle when patient tries to move
2	Moves, but not against gravity
3	Moves against gravity but not against resistance
4	Moves against resistance but not to full strength
5	Full strength (you cannot overcome the movement)

- Deep tendon, or muscle stretch, reflexes are tested with a patella hammer at the elbow to test biceps reflex initiated at the spinal level C5 and C6 and triceps reflex initiated at C7 and C8. The knee tendon is struck to assess the thigh muscle reflexes, initiated at L3 and L4. The Achilles tendon at the ankle is also tested.
- Superficial reflexes are initiated by receptors under the skin and can be elicited by stroking. These include abdominal reflexes, which are tested by stroking each side of the abdomen towards the umbilicus and below the umbilicus downwards. These reflexes may be disordered or absent in both upper and lower motor neurone disorders. Other reflexes in this group include corneal, gag, swallowing and perianal reflexes. Information about these reflexes may help nurses identify actual or potential problems in activities such as swallowing, micturating and defecating.
- Stroking the inner part of the sole tests plantar reflexes. The toes curl downwards in a normal response. If the toes extend or turn upwards, damage to the upper motor neurone is indicated (Fuller 1996).

Taking note of altered motor ability and the findings from assessment by other members of the team helps nurses to assess needs in the full range of activities, and promotes interdisciplinary working and purposeful interchange of clinical information (Kirrane 2000; Lehman *et al.* 2003).

ASSESSING BALANCE AND CO-ORDINATION

People with neurological damage may have lost the ability to sit unaided or without swaying, and they may have abnormal patterns of movement when moving from sitting to standing or when walking. Good co-ordination depends partly on the power of the muscles but also on the condition of the cerebellum. Mark, for example, lolls to one side when he is sitting, and as he walks his gait is unsteady, uneven and he bumps into things. He may have ataxia, a disorder of co-ordination, balance and rhythm caused by damage to his cerebellum sustained in the fight. Easily conducted estimates of balance and co-ordination integrity include the following:

- *Gait.* A wide based or unsteady gait (ataxia) may indicate cerebellar disease. This can be more obvious if the patient is unable to walk heel to toe.
- *Arms.* Ask the patient to touch the nurse's finger (which is held about 50 cm in front of the patient) with their index finger and then to quickly touch their own nose. Neurological problems may cause overshooting or tremor.
- *Legs.* Ask the patient to place one heel on the knee of the opposite leg and slowly slide the heel down the lower leg. This may reveal tremor or difficulty working out how to execute the movement.

Mark will also benefit from a thorough assessment by a physiotherapist.

THE ROLE OF THE PHYSIOTHERAPIST

Aspects of physiotherapy assessment can be a useful source of information for the nursing assessment. A physiotherapy assessment would include the following:

- *Posture and balance.* Assessment of this function would be able to inform assessment of the patient's need with regard to seating and support, mobility aids and level of supervision required
- *Range, strength and selectivity of voluntary movement, high or low muscle tone, range of joint movement.* Observations of these underpin the assessment of functional activities such as bed mobility, transfers, upper limb function, gait, and ability to use stairs. These inform nursing assessment of moving and handling needs, positioning in bed, positioning in a chair, use of wheelchair or mobility aids.
- *Sensory and perceptual function.* For example, some patients with Parkinson's disease may be able to use sensory stimulation such as rhythmic counting or rocking backwards and forwards or even using music to initiate movement.
- *Exercise tolerance and fatigue.* As nurses usually co-ordinate all aspects of a patient's care, information about how easily a person becomes fatigued can help nurses assess need for rest and activity.

- *Equipment options*. While nurses can assess the appropriate type of bed to use, physiotherapists can advise on therapeutic positioning needs, specialist seating, requirements or pressure relief options (Edwards 2002).

ASSESSING THE SENSORY SYSTEM

Nurses do not usually carry out a structured sensory assessment. However, assessment of patients' needs can be informed by using information recorded in the medical notes from a medical examination of sensory function. The sensory nerves supply distinct areas of the body, called dermatomes, and the sensory testing a doctor carries out includes the following:

- Pain – using a sensory testing needle.
- Temperature – with the patient's eyes closed and the flat forks of a tuning fork.
- Limb position – the thumb and large toe are moved up and down. The patient should be able to sense whether the movement is up or down.
- Vibration – with a vibrating tuning fork placed on the patient's sternum and bony prominence of big toe and thumb.
- Light touch – with the patient's eyes closed and a wisp of cotton wool.
- Two-point discrimination – with specific compasses and the patient's eyes closed.
- The special senses of sight, taste, hearing, smell.

Sensory disturbance occurs as tingling, numbness or hypersensitivity (also known as allodynia), where a normally non-painful stimulus is perceived as painful. Anwah (see case study in the section on How to Use this Book), may be suffering from disturbed sensory responses to the temperature of the water or the feel of shower droplets on her skin. This is common in conditions such as multiple sclerosis and other neuropathies. Louise (see case study) has altered sensation in her legs and may be prone to breaks in the skin caused by bumping against things. Exaggerated sensitivity can cause spasticity in a muscle through the action of reflex. Thus, a catheter bag, constipation, or sudden changes in environmental temperature can all act as 'noxious stimuli' that can cause a spastic response. Joyce (see case study) may have altered sensation or a hypersensitivity to bowel and bladder function that is making the spasticity in her lower body worse. Where there is no sensation, of course, the risks of injury and pressure damage is considerable. Ella (see case study) has altered sensation on her right side and is probably unable to perceive touch and pressure; consequently, she is at high risk of pressure damage on this side of her body.

Conscientious observation by nurses of a patient's verbal references to sensation and non-verbal responses to a changing sensory environment can help assess needs. Over time and with observation, Ella's weeping may be found to link with a factor in the environment. Nurses may notice that Miriam (see case study) has sensory deficits interfering with her swallowing, her ability to taste food or the ability to sense food in her mouth. Astute questioning and data collection can yield information on a greater number of variables than may be covered in conventional structured assessments. The identification of sensory deficits can help nurses assess needs in relation to self-care and vulnerability to injury.

THE ROLE OF THE OCCUPATIONAL THERAPIST
Assessment by an occupational therapist can produce useful, detailed clinical data on a patient's perceptual and cognitive functions. Occupational therapists will often use structured assessment tools that do this, such as the Rivermead test or the Chessington Occupational Therapy Neurological Assessment Battery (COTNAB). These tests generate information about a person's visual perception, object and face recognition, spatial ability, body image, memory, attention, and action, planning and sequencing. This involves evaluation of sensory discrimination, dexterity, co-ordination and the ability to follow written and spoken instructions – aspects that are discussed further in Chapter 11. However, the main disadvantages of these structured assessments are that they take place at one point in time and they have an element of 'the test' about them – a situation in which many of us may not perform well and which is outside a natural context. Nurses with good observation skills can

assess function in the course of their daily activities. After discussion with an occupational therapist, nurses can use their assessments of a patient's needs to facilitate activities such as washing and dressing, eating and drinking, eliminating, and working and playing (Kirrane 1999). Ongoing reassessment needs to be of abilities in these natural contexts.

AGNOSIA, APRAXIA AND COGNITIVE DEFICITS
Perceptual and cognitive assessment may include the following:

- Identification of *agnosia*, a perceptual disorder in which a person cannot identify an object despite the ability to recognise its tactile and visual elements (Grieve 1993). This would be important in assessing need with regard to the activity of washing and dressing, for example. In the case studies, a patient such as Miriam may in fact be experiencing a perceptual disturbance that makes it difficult for her to recognise utensils. Also, Mark may have a perceptual disorder that makes it difficult for him to perceive obstacles, and Harry may be unable to recognise faces.
- Identification of *apraxia*, where the person is unable to carry out purposeful, previously learned motor acts despite physical ability, willingness and an understanding of an instruction such as 'raise your right hand'. Again, Miriam may have some dyspraxia, which makes it difficult for her to plan how to set about picking up a knife and fork. Also, as Ella's recovery progresses and she becomes more mobile, it may become clear that she has some dyspraxia.
- Identification of disorders of attention, concentration, memory and orientation, problem solving. Any acquired brain injury can produce deficits in any of these areas. Harry, for example, clearly has some problems with orientation and memory, and this seems to compound his emotional distress; this could also be true of Miriam, Ella, Gary and Anwah.
- Identification of other aspects of physical functioning may also affect self-care and daily living skills, such as fine motor control and hand functions (Reed 2001). Louise and Irene, for example, are primarily affected in the lower part of their bodies, but evaluation of hand and arm control may have

important implications for needs assessment in the other activities of living. Fred too may have upper limb limitation, and Ella will certainly have reduced grip on her affected side.

THE ROLE OF THE SPEECH AND LANGUAGE THERAPIST

Nurses usually assess communication ability informally through interaction and can sometimes carry out a swallowing screen if there are concerns about swallowing function. Training to carry out a bedside swallowing evaluation is often provided by a speech and language therapist. These issues are discussed more fully in Chapter 4. Full assessment by a speech and language therapist establishes a thorough evaluation of the cranial nerves involved in swallowing, speaking and breathing, and also assesses language processing and production in the cerebral lobes. The assessment of communication and swallowing needs can inform the nursing assessment and provide clinical grounds to help prioritise communication needs throughout all activities, particularly in relation to eating and drinking. Communication and swallowing deficits are very common following a brain injury, particularly stroke, and Ella's assessment could show deficits in these areas.

MAIN DIAGNOSTIC AND INVESTIGATIVE PROCEDURES

In addition to the physical and psychological assessment by the multidisciplinary team, a further source of information for nursing assessment is the results of tests and diagnostic investigations carried out by radiographers, laboratory technicians, and neurophysiologists. The main tests and investigations are summarised in Table 2.2.

PSYCHOLOGICAL WELL-BEING OF PATIENT AND FAMILY

Neurological damage often brings about major changes in a person's lifestyle and independence, affecting the emotional well-being of patients, families and close friends (Connelly and Bidwell 2001). A sudden major traumatic event or the cumulative effect of stresses in long-term disability can overwhelm the coping strategies of the people involved. Nurse assessment needs to include the following:

Table 2.2 Common neurological tests and investigations.

Test or investigation	Purpose
Angiography (cerebral)	To detect aneurysm, arterio-venous malformation, vasospasm, rupture or interrupted blood flow
CT scan	To detect thrombus, intracranial bleed, tumours, tissue shift
Digital subtraction angiography	Helps to visualise blood flow and detect hydrocephalus, vascular abnormalities such as aneurysm or haematoma
Electroencephalography (EEG)	To detect abnormal patterns of neuronal electrical activity as in seizure activity
Electromyography	Differentiates between peripheral nerve and muscle disorders
Evoked potentials	To detect neurological problems of vision, hearing, mixed nerves of hand and leg
Lumbar puncture	To remove some spinal fluid to look for micro-organisms, blood cells, tumour markers and chemical changes
Magnetic resonance imaging (MRI)	Can detect changes caused by hypoxia, necrosis, degenerative disease, tumour and haematoma. Gives clearer picture than CT scan
Myelography	To detect blockage of spinal cord
Neuropsychological evaluation	To evaluate perception, spatial ability, memory, action planning and sequencing, mood and behaviour
Full blood count	Can indicate illness underlying non-specific neurological symptoms or deficiency leading to neuropathy
Other tests	Can show blood clotting or deficiency which may cause stroke, peripheral neuropathy, confusion, vasculitis
Urea and electrolytes, creatinine, glucose	Can show abnormalities which may cause confusion, delirium, neuropathy, coma

- The family's perceptions of and reactions to the situation.
- The needs of the people involved who may have high anxiety levels and stress levels or depression.
- The opportunities for counselling and the extent to which the needs can be met by nurses or whether to refer to other professionals. The most important factor for people with

neurological conditions is being able to access health professionals who have a good understanding of their needs. The key is to refer to specialist units and services as promptly as possible (Neurological Alliance 2001, 2003).

• How much information the patient and family require and the support groups that can help them.

As indicated in Chapter 1, the interaction of physical and psychological states can be strong. The impact of good emotional and psychological support on the sense of well-being of patients with long-term conditions, can be as effective as physical treatment.

SUMMARY

❏ Assessment of level of consciousness, scored using the Glasgow Coma Scale, to detect changes of alertness indicated by eye opening, motor response of limbs to verbal or painful stimuli, verbal orientation to time, place and person. Temperature, respiration rate and depth, pulse rate, blood pressure, particularly for warning signs of rising intracranial pressure.

❏ Estimating pupil size, reactivity, shape and equality in response to light.

❏ Evaluating motor ability by assessing the patient's limb power, balance and co-ordination, ability to move spontaneously, and to swallow safely and the effect on the activities of living.

❏ Evaluation of sensory function, particularly in relation to pain, pressure and temperature, and the effect on self-care abilities.

❏ Integrating nursing assessment of altered cognition, altered motor ability and altered sensation with assessment, tests and investigations by members of the interdisciplinary team to develop integrated care planning.

❏ Assessment of the psychological needs of the patient and their family in acute or longer-term neurological illness, drawing on support from other professionals and self-help organisations.

REFERENCES

Connolly, C. E. and Bidwell, A. S. (2001) Affiliative relationships phenomena. In Stewart-Amidei, C. and Kunkel, J. A. (eds) *AANN's Neuroscience Nursing: Human Responses to Neurologic Dysfunction*, 2nd edn. W. B. Saunders, New York, chapter 16.

Edwards, S. (2002) *Neurological Physiotherapy*, 2nd edn. Churchill Livingstone, Edinburgh.

Edwards, S. L. (2001) Using the Glasgow Coma Scale: analysis and limitations. *British Journal of Nursing* **10**, 2.

Fairley, D. and Cosgrove, J. (1999) Glasgow Coma Scale: improving nursing practice through clinical effectiveness. *Nursing in Critical Care* **4** (6), 276–9.

Frawley, P. (1990) Neurological observations. *Nursing Times* **86** (35), 29–34.

Fuller, G. (1996) *Neurological Examination Made Easy*. Churchill Livingstone, Edinburgh.

Grieve, J. (1993) *Neuropsychology for Occupational Therapists*. Blackwell Science, Oxford.

Hickey, J. (1997) *The Clinical Practice of Neurological and Neurosurgical Nursing*, 4th edn. Lippincott, Philadelphia.

Jevon, P. and Ewens, B. (2002) *Monitoring the Critically Ill Patient*. Blackwell Science, Oxford.

Juarez, J. and Lyons, M. (1995) Interrater reliability of the Glasgow Coma Scale. *Journal of Neuroscience Nursing* **27** (5), 283–6.

Kirrane, C. (2000) Evidence-based practice in neurology: a team approach to development. *Nursing Standard* **14** (52), 43–5.

Lehman, C. A., Hayes, J. M., LeCroix, M., Owen, S. V. and Nauta, J. W. (2003) Development and implementation of a problem focussed neurological assessment. *Journal of Neuroscience Nursing* **35** (4), 185–92.

Lower, J. (1992) Rapid neuro assessment. *American Journal of Nursing* **92** (6), 38–45.

Neurological Alliance (2001) *Levelling Up Standards of Care for People with a Neurological Condition*. The Neurological Alliance, London.

Neurological Alliance (2003) *In Search of a Service*. Neurological Alliance, London.

NICE (National Institute for Clinical Excellence) (2002) *Head Injury Guidelines*. HMSO, London.

Reed, K. L. (2001) *Quick Reference Guide to Occupational Therapy*, 2nd edn. Aspen, Maryland.

Rowley, G. and Fielding, K. (1991) Reliability and accuracy of the Glasgow Coma Scale with experienced and inexperienced users. *Lancet* **337**, 535–8.

Shah, S. (1999) Neurological assessment. *Nursing Standard* **13** (22), 49–55.

Stewart-Amidei, C. and Kunkel, J. A. (eds) (2001) *AANN's Neuroscience Nursing: Human Responses to Neurologic Dysfunction*, 2nd edn. W. B. Saunders, New York.

Teasdale, G. and Jennet, B. (1974) Assessment of coma and impaired consciousness. *Lancet* **2**, 81–4.

Woodrow, P. (2000) Head injuries: acute care. *Nursing Standard* **14** (35), 37–44.

3 | Maintaining a Safe Environment

INTRODUCTION

The ability to keep oneself safe is a blend of learned behaviour, reflex action and homeostatic adjustment that is often compromised in neurological patients. They may be prone to falls and pressure sores or to loss of the protective reflexes such as blinking and swallowing because of motor problems. Warning sensations such as pain, hot or cold, may be lost because of reduced sensation or perceptual deficits, and impaired perception and cognition reduce reasoning ability and judgement about safe choices and appropriate actions to keep safe. One of the most difficult aspects of planning safe care lies in balancing the patient's rights, risks, safety and autonomy. The aims of this chapter are to describe a range of assessment tools that can be used to help plan safe care and to describe a range of possible interventions.

LEARNING OUTCOMES

❏ Discuss the management of a patient in pain, with specific attention to neuropathic pain.

❏ Discuss the principles of pressure sore risk assessment and prevention in patients with altered sensation and altered mobility.

❏ Differentiate the meaning of the terms wandering, confusion, motor restlessness, seizure activity, and spasticity, and choose appropriate interventions to foster a safe environment.

❏ Describe the nursing assessment and risk management of patients with altered cognition, impaired spatial awareness, agnosia and apraxia.

❏ Discuss the role of the interdisciplinary team in risk management and maintaining a safe environment.

❏ Outline the ethical and professional issues arising in risk management.

ALTERED SENSATION: PAIN

The International Association for the Study of Pain defines pain as an unpleasant sensory and emotional experience with actual or potential tissue damage or one that is described in such terms (Inbody 1998). When the sensation of pain first arises, a person will also feel anxious. Fears arise in the mind about what is causing the pain, whether it will get worse and whether it is serious or life threatening. The person may eventually worry enough to seek help, particularly since the high anxiety levels worsen the pain experience (Ricci and Barker 1994; Axford and O'Callaghan 2004).

Types of pain

Acute pain is protective and warns of an injury or insult. It may be time limited and resolved completely or it may go on to become chronic. Treatment aims to eradicate the underlying cause and control the pain by appropriate drugs, such as opioids or anti-inflammatory drugs. Table 3.1 shows examples

Table 3.1 Actions of analgesics.

Drug	Actions and uses
Aspirin and aspirin-like drugs	Inhibit the release of the chemical prostaglandin which stimulates the nociceptors. Contraindicated for patients who have had a cerebral bleed
Non-steroidal anti-inflammatory medication	Also damp down inflammation by inhibiting prostaglandin release. Useful in conditions affecting muscle, bones and joints
Steroids	Suppress inflammation, allergic reactions and immune system activity
Opioids	Depress activity in the central nervous system
Anticonvulsants (can be used to alleviate neuropathic pain)	Inhibit brain cells and damp down electrical activity in neurones
Antidepressants (can be used to alleviate neuropathic pain)	Affect neurotransmitter levels and neuronal activity

of drugs commonly used to treat pain. In addition, non-invasive measures may be used such as application of heat or cold, manipulation, splinting, transcutaneous electrical nerve stimulation, or relaxation therapy to reduce anxiety and body tension as shown in Table 3.2.

Chronic pain is pain that has lasted continuously or intermittently over time, usually one to three months. Inbody (1998) suggests that pain can be regarded as chronic if it

- persists for one month beyond the usual course of an acute illness or healing injury;
- is associated with a chronic pathological process; or
- recurs at intervals of months or years.

By this time, if a diagnosis has been made, the patient may acknowledge that pain is part of their life and may become depressed rather than anxious. The treatment is similar to that

Table 3.2 Non-pharmacological pain management.

Intervention	Possible uses
Heat therapy	Increases blood flow and removal of waste products, relaxes muscle tone. Use cautiously with patients with sensory loss or circulatory problems
Cold therapy	Causes vasoconstriction and decreased nerve conduction, reduces oedema and bleeding. Use with caution in patients with reduced sensation or circulatory problems
Massage	Stimulates peripheral receptors that send pleasurable messages to the brain. Caution in patients with multiple sclerosis.
Range of movement exercises	Decrease muscle tension, spasticity and contracture; increase strength and endurance
Transcutaneous electrical stimulation	Stimulates cutaneous nerve endings by small electric current. These compete with pain messages. Not to be used in patients with heart disease, pacemakers or no sensation
Relaxation, breathing exercises and visualisation	Reduce anxiety levels, lower muscle tone and pacify the autonomic nervous system

of acute pain, but with a much greater emphasis on developing effective coping strategies such as breathing and muscle relaxation, self-hypnosis and visualisation, distraction, self-help and support groups. In addition, counselling can help alleviate depression often associated with this kind of pain.

Classification of pain

There are three major categories of pain defined by the underlying pathophysiology. *Nociceptive* pain means the sensation of something harmful or injurious in the tissues of the body. It is caused by stimulation of nociceptors that are located at the site of tissue injury. Just as mechanoreceptors detect touch, pressure, vibration and stretch, thermoreceptors respond to temperature, chemoreceptors respond to solutions, tastes, smells and changes in blood chemistry, and photoreceptors respond to light, so nociceptors respond to pain. Some textbooks do differ in their views on how different receptors can respond to pain. Marieb (1992) suggests that any type of stimulus, if applied vigorously, can cause pain, although Carroll and Bowsher (1993) assert that pain can never result from overstimulation of sensation-specific nerve endings. Whatever the physiology, nociceptive pain occurs when receptors respond to irritation from excess heat or cold, excess pressure, vibration, stretch or corrosive substances. Pain messages follow the sensory pathways dedicated to noxious stimuli. The pain is often worse on movement. Joyce (see case study in the section on How to Use this Book), is probably suffering some pain from her arthritic knee, which may have worsened and stiffened because of her reduced mobility since her accident. There may be swelling in the knee and signs of inflammation, which all indicate a nociceptive-type pain. She may also be experiencing a cramping type of pain from excess muscle contraction and spasticity.

By contrast, *neuropathic pain* arises from damage to the neurones themselves. The damaged neurones are irritable, unstable, can initiate signals without involving specific pain receptors in the tissues and can also produce an exaggerated response to receptor stimulation. Thus, a normally painless experience, such as being touched or breathing air through an open mouth, can be experienced as painful. This is called *allodynia*. A study by

Widor *et al.* (2002) found that cold was the factor most increasing neuropathic pain following a stroke. There may also be an exaggerated pain response, called *hyperalgesia*, to stimuli such as incontinence or to discomfort from the sensation of catheter bags. Hyperalgesia may cause painful muscle spasms or trigger spasticity in neurological patients. The burning sensation that Louise (see case study in the section on How to Use this Book) has in her legs is neuropathic. The myelin damage to the sensory neurones is causing abnormal conduction and consequently abnormal sensation. It could also manifest as hypersensitivity to touch, such as not liking the feel of the bedclothes on her legs. Neuropathic pain can also be caused by damage to the thalamus. Anwah (see case study) has extensive cerebral damage, and quite possibly damage to the thalamus, making her hypersensitive to the rapid changes of temperature that take place in washing and dressing with reduced homeostatic responses.

Pain descriptors

Patients who are able to communicate their sensations of pain verbally may describe neuropathic pain as shooting, lancinating or burning whereas nociceptive pain might be described as throbbing, pressing or aching. Both types of pain can occur alone or together (Wilson 2002). Post-stroke pain, for example, can be neuropathic because it arises from damage to the thalamus and nociceptive because it arises from a shoulder joint (RCP 1999). Ella (see case study) could well be experiencing both 'thalamic' or 'central pain' and nociceptive pain from a badly positioned shoulder, for example.

Causes of neuropathic pain

Neuropathic pain can also be experienced spontaneously from damage to neurones in the central or peripheral nerves caused by the following:

- Trauma or surgery – patients who have had a limb amputation may experience phantom pain which is a type of neuropathic pain.
- Ischaemia because of vascular disease causing damage to receptors in tissues.

- Infections such as herpes or cellulitis, or post-viral infections such as shingles or trigeminal neuralgia, which causes direct inflammation of sensory neurones.
- Degenerative nerve changes such as in multiple sclerosis or diabetic neuropathy where the neurones are damaged by demyelination.
- Post-stroke pain because of vascular injury to parts of the thalamus, which is an important part of sensory processing. This is called thalamic or central pain (Inbody 1998).

Management of neuropathic pain

Because neuropathic (also called neurogenic) pain does not involve nociceptive receptors it does not follow normal pain pathways and does not respond to the opioids or anti-inflammatory analgesia used to control the pain of damaged tissue. Management of neurogenic pain aims to pacify neuronal conduction and transmission. It includes:

- antidepressants;
- anticonvulsants;
- non-pharmacological methods such as relaxation, breathing exercises, visualisation, counselling, heat and cold therapy, complementary therapies or transcutaneous electrical stimulation.

Psychosomatic or psychogenic pain

The term *psychosomatic* refers to a concept that cuts across the division of diseases into physical (somatic) and mental (psycho). It is generally used to describe a sensation of pain for which organic cause cannot be found or for which the pain experience is disproportionate to the cause. Psychosomatic pain is sometimes regarded as conscious or unconscious manipulative behaviour by which a sufferer derives secondary gains from the attention that the pain experience generates. Others regard it as a high state of arousal in the nervous system, such as anxiety or tension, that produces physical symptoms such as pain. If an organic cause cannot be found, counselling and psychotherapy may help reduce this kind of pain experience.

Pain assessment

Although it is not possible to measure pain objectively, nurses can use a range of techniques to assess pain and evaluate pain management interventions.

- Assessment and monitoring of visual indicators, physiological and physical manifestations.
- Patients self-report on the location, quality, intensity, duration, pattern, associated factors and alleviation of pain.
- Report of parent, family or others close to the patient.
- Use of a suitable pain tool or chart.

Pain assessment tools

There is a variety of pain assessment and pain relief tools that use different strategies to assess pain experience. These include visual analogue scales, numerical rating scales, verbal rating scales, faces pain scale, pain thermometer scales and the McGill pain questionnaire. Evaluations of pain assessment tools (Baillie 1993; Ho *et al.* 1996; Lawler 1997; Bird 2003) indicate that no one tool has robust reliability and validity in all patient populations and that patients with cognitive disturbances present particular difficulties. Table 3.3 shows a comparison of a range of different tools.

In choosing a tool, the following points need to be considered (Carroll and Bowsher 1993).

- Choose a simple tool that is quick and easy to use, but that has been validated and shown to work.
- Try out a selection of charts to find the one that is the most suitable, and adapt it if possible to meet the needs of patients with communication or cognitive problems.
- Ensure that those who are to use the tool – nurses, patients and carers – understand them.
- Find out from other users what they think – pros and cons.
- Make sure that assessment and evaluation are done regularly.
- Act promptly on the results shown from the assessment.

The literature recognises that cognitive impairment makes the use of pain measurement tools problematical (Ferrell *et al.* 1995; Krulewitch 2000; Delac 2002), and that patients with an altered

Table 3.3 Examples of pain assessment tools (Bird 2003, reproduced with permission from Nursing Standard).

Tool	Use with older patients	Use with patients who are cognitively impaired	Translation and multicultural use
Visual analogue scale	■ Valid tool if self-completion is appropriate ■ Careful instruction and presentation required ■ The nurse can assist completion but bias may be introduced ■ Visual impairment may affect accuracy of results ■ Of the tools discussed here, this is the most sensitive to small changes in pain intensity	■ Low completion rate found in this population ■ Careful instruction and presentation required ■ Nurse can assist completion but bias may be introduced ■ Visual impairment may affect accuracy of results	■ Easily translated as only anchor descriptors and instruction required ■ Successfully used in Italian and French ■ Appropriate for cross-cultural study
Numeric rating scale	■ Appropriate if patient can translate pain into numbers ■ Careful explanation and presentation required ■ Sensitive to intensity changes but less so than VAS	■ Few in this group could perceive pain as numbers ■ Other tools are more appropriate ■ Verbal administration alone is not enough	■ Appropriate for cross-cultural study as numbers are not subject to translation error ■ Patient comprehension should be ensured. Can the patient understand pain as a number?

Table 3.3 *Continued*

Tool	Use with older patients	Use with patients who are cognitively impaired	Translation and multicultural use
Verbal rating scale	■ Wording requires careful selection ■ Asking how pain has changed since the last assessment may enhance results ■ Not as sensitive as VAS or NRS but too many descriptors can be confusing ■ High completion rates ■ Can be verbally administered	■ High completion rate ■ Can be verbally administered ■ Lacks the sensitivity of other scales	■ Ease of translation depends on target language, but has been successful in Italian ■ Cross-cultural study appropriate once the translation is validated ■ A greater number of descriptors may cause greater error in translation
Faces pain scale	■ Clear instruction and presentation required ■ Visual difficulties can prevent completion ■ High completion rates within this group	■ Low completion rate when modified version used ■ Can be valuable with careful presentation and assessment of patient ability	■ Translation is not required as pictorial ■ Could be used in cross-cultural study but no evidence of this as yet ■ Versatile – useful where a translated tool is required but not available

McGill pain questionnaire	■ Communication difficulties directly affect completion ■ Shortened version more appropriate if patients cannot tolerate lengthy assessment and Illustrations may assist the patient to understand the descriptors ■ Shortened version more appropriate	■ Validity not confirmed in this patient group	■ Translation complicated due to descriptors ■ A translation may be useful in the target population once validated but cross-cultural comparison is inappropriate
Brief pain inventory	■ Data suggests limited clinical use but valid tool ■ Shortened version more appropriate if patients cannot tolerate lengthy assessment	■ Difficult to use with this patient population ■ Higher degrees of cognitive impairment associated with higher rates of non-completion	■ Already used for cross-cultural study as validated in various languages ■ Translated copies could be obtained for self-completion by the patient ■ Could be successfully used by translator
Non-verbal pain measures	■ Selection available but none highly accurate as behavioural interpretation is subjective ■ Checklist of non-verbal pain indicators correlates highly with VRS and may be used together where patient's level of consciousness is likely to change ■ Not completely reliable as behaviour can be interpreted in varying ways	■ No one tool holds particularly high stability in testing but the checklist of non-verbal pain indicators was developed specifically for use with this group	■ Patient comprehension not required but instructions require clear translation ■ DOLOPLUS 2 scale, originally in French, is being validated in other language versions and is the most appropriate for cross-cultural study ■ Pain behaviour varies within cultures and between cultures so caution is advised when interpreting results

consciousness level or cognitive impairment are less likely to be diagnosed with pain (RCP 1999). The difficulty has prompted greater interest in the use of non-verbal pain indicators (Feldt 2000; Delac 2002). For patients with an altered level of consciousness or impaired verbal communication there is a high reliance on the interpretation of these bodily and behavioural clues (see Tables 3.4–3.6). The nursing team need to discuss the indicators as they occur spontaneously or while care is being delivered to try to detect an emerging pattern. Anwah, for example, would clearly be unable to participate in using an

Table 3.4 Non-verbal signs of pain.

Body and behaviour	Signs
Body movements	Abnormal posture, guarding body part, avoiding use of body part, restlessness, high muscle tone, exaggerated response to normal touch, violence or non-cooperation in care delivery
Facial	Unusually frequent or infrequent eye contact, tears, grimacing
Vocal	Change of vocal pitch, tone, pace and fluency; sobbing, groaning, high-pitched calls and noises, abnormal quietness
Interaction	Attention seeking, withdrawal
Emotion	Anxiety, anger, aggression

Table 3.5 Physiological and physical indicators of pain.

Indicator	Signs
Physiological signs (to be interpreted cautiously as these may be influenced by other physical and emotional states)	Relative changes in blood pressure, respiration rate and pulse (particularly important in people with actual or potential intracranial problems), change in temperature indicating infection
Physical	Muscle wasting, muscle spasms, change in temperature of skin, signs of swelling, reddening or skin irritation

Table 3.6 Common neurological conditions and pain.

Condition	Pain type	Potential cause
Stroke	Nociceptive	From badly positioned limbs or poor manual handling causing tissue or joint damage, very often in the shoulder joint. Current guidelines suggest this is more likely than subluxation due to stroke (RCP 1999)
	Neuropathic pain; 'central pain' or thalamic pain	Pain arising from thalamus following stroke. May arise spontaneously or may over-respond to sensory stimuli
Sub-arachnoid haemorrhage	Nociceptive and neuropathic	Headache due to bleeding causing pressure on pain-sensitive structures and to ischaemia caused by vasospasm
Multiple sclerosis	Neuropathic	Hypersensitivity to temperature and touch due to demyelination
Traumatic brain injury	Nociceptive and neuropathic	The brain itself is insensitive to pain. Pain arises from traction, pressure, displacement, inflammation or dilatation of pain-sensitive structures such as the scalp, head and neck muscles, blood vessels and some of the cranial nerves
Headache	Nociceptive or neuropathic depending on cause	May be caused by cerebral vasodilation, ischaemia, intracranial pressure or infection, substance withdrawal, cranial neuralgias
Guillain-Barré	Neuropathic	Pain in limbs caused by inflammation of peripheral nerves
Spinal cord injury/damage	Nociceptive and neuropathic	Neuronal trauma, degeneration or pressure
Trigeminal neuralgia	Neuropathic	Severe, paroxysmal pain in the face following the path of the trigeminal nerve
Diabetic neuropathy	Nociceptive and neuropathic and chronic	Ischaemia, damage to neurone because of excess glucose

interactive tool, but nurses could develop an observation scheme based on non-verbal responses to assess her pain experience and evaluate the effectiveness of pain relief measures.

Interventions

The rationale for most interventions is based on the 'gate control' theory of pain (Wall and Melzack 1999). This suggests that neuronal activity in the spinal cord can increase or suppress the transmission of nociception to the brain; for example, modifying activity in the brain with opioids or psychotherapy 'pushes' the gate closed from above by interrupting pain signals that arrive at the spinal cord. Massage, transcutaneous electrical stimulation and anti-inflammatory medication 'pull' the gate closed from below by acting on the pain receptors and interfering with the pain signal at receptor level. The pain experience can be relieved and modified by planning care that takes into account pharmacological, non-invasive physical means and psychotherapeutic techniques. Louise, for example, has a lot of stress in her life, and while the steroid treatment to control her flare-up will help control the pain in her legs, techniques to help her manage her stress, counselling and distraction will lessen the pain experience because her body will be less tense.

Interdisciplinary care planning is valuable in planning and evaluating pain management so that patients can comfortably participate in physiotherapy, occupational therapy and speech and language therapies, and are as alert and as attentive as possible. In addition, pain management guidelines are constantly being updated as new research on the effectiveness of treatment emerges. The Cochrane database has regular updates and it is important to keep abreast of these changes by visiting the website. For example, the pain management guidelines for the prevention and management of shoulder pain in stroke patients (RCP 2002) suggests the following:

- avoid overhead arm slings;
- use foam supports;
- educate staff about correct handling.

If pain has already developed, recommended treatment suggests:

- start with simple interventions such as non steroidal anti-inflammatory drugs;
- use high-intensity transcutaneous electrical stimulation (TENS).

Most charities and support groups that deal with specific neurological diseases are able to offer a wealth of research evidence and management guidelines, and readers are strongly recommended to consult these regularly. Contact information is given in Appendix 1.

Evaluation

Evaluation of the success of pain management will depend on whether the pain is acute or chronic, the level of control anticipated and how far the patient is able to participate in planning goals, interventions and evaluations. Table 3.7 gives some examples of potential pain factors in a range of different neurological conditions. Ongoing monitoring can help to establish patterns of pain control related to therapy, reassessment using pain assessment tools, discussion with patient, and evaluation of bodily and non-verbal responses while the patient is carrying out normal activities of living. With Joyce, for example, the pain from her osteoarthritis is chronic and the goal would need to reflect the level of pain control that can be achieved. For Louise, however, the neuropathic sensation of burning in her legs may completely resolve when the treatment for her disease allows her some remission, or remain at a sub-acute level. If pain management measures are unsatisfactory, there should be a full reassessment, including a thorough evaluation of the source and type of pain.

RISK OF PRESSURE SORES, INJURIES AND FALLS

Patients with a neurological impairment can quickly develop pressure sores, skin abrasions or burns because of reduced sensation and movement. They are also at greater risk for falls or injury, not only because of neurological deficits, but also because they may suffer some of the side effects of the drug treatments for the condition. Examples of these are shown in Table 3.8.

Table 3.7 Conditions and specific risk factors.

	Altered motor ability	Altered sensation	Altered perception	Specific pain factors
Stroke	Hemiplegia and weakness Spasticity Poor balance	Lack of proprioception Loss of sensation	Impaired judgement of depth and distance Route-finding problems Apraxia and agnosia	Central or thalamic pain Shoulder pain
Dementia	Loss of co-ordination	Misinterpretation of stimuli	Misinterpretation Loss of memory	Inability to communicate pain experience
Parkinson's disease	Tremor Rigidity Immobility Postural instability	May hallucinate because of medication or may develop hypotension	Drug psychosis and confusion with delusions Dementia may occur in later stages	Cramping pains due to overstretched muscles and tendons
Multiple sclerosis	Fatigue Spasticity Weakness Impaired balance and posture	Hypersensitivity with allodynia	Depression Memory loss Reasoning, information processing, attention and concentration may be impaired	Neuropathic pain Nociceptive pain
Epilepsy	Seizure activity and altered consciousness	During seizure may not be aware of sensation	During seizure may not be aware of external environment	Potential for injury in seizure activity May be mistaken for wandering or confusion
Traumatic brain injury	Fatigue Spasticity Weakness Impaired balance and posture	Impairment or loss of sensation depending on site of brain injury	Reduced level of consciousness initially Agnosia, apraxia, loss of topographical orientation	Neuropathic or central pain

Table 3.8 Side effects of medication and safety risk.

Condition	Medication	Possible risk from side effect
Parkinson's disease	Selegeline	Confusion, falls due to autonomic disturbance and hypotension
	COMT inhibitor	May increase dyskinesia
	Anticholinergics	Causes confusion and not to be used with elderly patients
	Levodopa	Hypotension and risk of falls Confusion in elderly patients
	Dopamine agonists	Hallucinations, delusions, confusion
	Amantidine	Psychosis
Multiple scleorsis	Baclofen	Weakness, drowsiness, dizziness
	Diazepam	Drowsiness and dizziness
Epilepsy	Benzodiazepines	Sedation, dizziness, fatigue
	Carbamezepine	Diplopia, dizziness
	Ethosuximide	Dizziness
	Gabapentin	Dipopia, dizziness, sedation, tremor
	Lamotrigine	Drowsiness, dizziness, headache
	Phenobarbitone	Sedation, fatigue, cognitive impairment
	Phenytoin	Blurred vision, dizziness, unsteadiness, impaired cognitive function, headache
	Sodium valproate	Tremor, drowsiness
	Vigabatrin	Dizziness, sedation
Stroke	Antidepressants, amitriptyline	Drowsiness or decreased alertness
	Anticonvulsants (see epilepsy)	Weakness or floppiness
	Antispasticity medication	
Alzheimer's disease	Sedatives	Decreased awareness

Altered sensation: pressure sores, injury and falls

Sensation may be impaired and the patient may not have sensory experience of pressure. Patients may not be aware of the warning signs of reduced blood flow, such as pins and needles, or of the painful sensation of a break in the skin, or of skin irritation from other noxious stimuli such as catheters, nasogastric tubes or the presence of urine or faeces on the skin. Sensory deficits have been shown to be one of the most important factors in pressure sore risk assessments (Halfens *et al.* 2000), and the impairment should be identified in the neurological assessment.

In addition, there could be *altered proprioception*. Proprioceptors are special receptors located in muscles and tendons that carry messages to the brain about where the limb is in relation to the body. Patients may be unaware that a limb is dangling, that they are lying on it or that it is trapped in an awkward position.

Patients may also have visual field deficits, such as hemianopia, blurred or double vision, tunnel vision, or they may have reduced spatial awareness, finding it difficult to judge distances or differentiate an object from its background (Grieve 1993). Mark (see case study in the section on How to Use this Book) may have some visual impairment following his assault, or there may be some disturbance in proprioception, both of which could be causing him to bump into things.

Altered motor ability

Altered motor ability can take the form of reduced mobility, immobility, restlessness or repetitiveness, and excessive or reduced muscle tone leading to the risk of pressure sore damage, muscle weakness, spasticity, fatigue and instability in sitting or while walking.

Reduced mobility or immobility

Motor pathway damage restricts a person's ability to alter their position independently. Some patients may experience sensory discomfort, but are unable to express the discomfort, or unable to work out how to relieve the discomfort. Both Anwah and Ella are at risk in this way. Patients with Parkinson's disease have an increased risk of falling not only because of slow reflexes but also because the anti-Parkinson medications may cause postural hypertension and involuntary movements (Gray and Hildebrand 2000; Calne and Kumar 2003). Fred (see case study) is particularly at risk in this way, especially as his medication management is not yet stable. Patients who have suffered an acquired brain injury may have hemiplegia that alters mobility and balance. Ella could initially be nursed in a profiling bed with fixed bed rails to maintain her safety, if indicated by assessment. This should be explained to her using pointing and gesture if necessary to obtain her permission. It should also be established whether Ella was a smoker before her stroke as she may be suffering withdrawal symptoms of restlessness and discomfort that could be relieved by the use of nicotine patches.

Motor restlessness and repetitive movements

Some types of neurological impairment result in restless or repetitive movements that can lead to shearing or friction damage to the skin. Patients may repeatedly move a leg up and down the bed resulting in friction damage to the heel; they may pluck at parts of their body or equipment resulting in skin damage over time; or they may cause friction damage to the head and ears from repetitive head movements. Restlessness in bed or getting in and out of bed without an apparent purpose, or for a purpose that the person is unable to communicate, may indicate *seizure activity*. This can involve fumbling with bedclothes or taking clothes off, for no apparent reason. Harry (see case study) may be particularly at risk of friction forces on his skin, personal injury from his plucking activity and may be at further risk of falling if the restlessness is due to seizure activity and he is experiencing altered awareness levels.

Altered muscle tone

Patients may develop uneven muscle tone resulting in painful spasticity that can go on to develop into a *contracture*. Arms, legs or fingers may become rigid in *flexion* and sores may develop in the acute angle between the two contracted joints. Joyce is particularly at risk if her spasticity remains untreated. Other patients may have reduced muscle tone that makes the limbs and body *flaccid*, which is common in the early days after a stroke. There is additional risk from weakness, postural sway, altered sitting balance and fatigue. Other neurological conditions such as multiple sclerosis and motor neurone disease cause alterations in muscle tone. Both Irene (see case study) and Louise have lowered leg muscle tone, and the muscles may fatigue easily.

Pressure sore risk and prevention

A general neurological assessment will identify the deficits that contribute to pressure sore risk, and several risk assessment scales exist to supplement this (Hamilton 1992; Flanagan 1993; Wall 2000; NICE 2003c; Waters and Anderson 2003). Figure 3.1 shows an example. However, current recommendations are that while risk assessment scales are useful they should only be used as an aide-memoire and should not replace clinical judgement (RCN 2000; Rycroft-Malone 2000, Rycroft-Malone and McInness 2000) and where possible be validated for use in neurological patients. Clinical judgement involves the whole interdisciplinary team, requiring each member to take responsibility for sharing care and expertise. Examples of how different neurological conditions may affect sensation and motor ability are shown in Table 3.7. Physiotherapists in particular can advise on suitable positioning and some types of pressure-relieving equipment, and these are discussed in more detail in the chapter on mobilising.

Pressure sore risk assessment (RCN 2000; DoH 2001; NICE 2003a, c)

- Identify individuals 'at risk' using clinical judgement, risk assessment scale and members of the interdisciplinary team.
- Key risk factors include reduced mobility, reduced sensation, acute illness, altered level of consciousness, age, previous history of pressure sores. Neurological conditions are recognised as posing particular risk.
- Previous history of pressure damage.
- Vascular disease.
- Severe chronic or terminal illness.
- Malnutrition.
- Medications such as sedatives, hypnotics, analgesics, anti-inflammatories.

Risk Assessment Tool – Pressure Ulcer Prevention

Patient's Name:	Hospital No:

Waterlow Pressure Sore Prevention/Treatment Policy

Ring scores in table, add total. Several scores per category can be used

Build/Weight for Height	★	Skin Type Visual Risk Areas	★	Sex Age	★	Special Risks	★
						Tissue Malnutrition	★
Average	0	Healthy	0	Male	1	e.g.: Terminal Cachexia	8
(BMI 20–24.9)		Tissue paper	1	Female	2	Cardiac Failure	5
Above Average		Dry	1	14–49	1	Peripheral Vascular	
(BMI 25–30.9)	1	Oedematous	1	50–64	2	Disease	5
Obese		Clammy (Temp ↑)	1	65–74	3	Anaemia	2
(BMI >30.9)	2	Discoloured	2	75–80	4	Smoking	1
Below Average		Broken/Spot	3	81+	5		
(BMI <20)	3						
Continence	★	**Mobility**	★	**Appetite**	★	**Neurological Deficit**	★
Complete/		Fully	0	Usual		e.g. Diabetes, MS, CVA,	
Catheterised	0	Restless/Fidgety	1	Appetite	0	Motor/Sensory	
Occasion incont	1	Apathetic	2	Reduced		Paraplegia	4-6
Cath/incontinent		Restricted	3	Appetite	1		
of faeces	2	Inert/Traction	4	NG Tube/			
Doubly incont	3	Chairbound	5	fluids only	2		
				NBM/Not			
				eating			
				Anorexic	3		

						Major Surgery/Trauma	★
						Orthopaedic –	
Score	**10+** At Risk	**15+** High Risk	**20+** Very High Risk			Below waist, spinal	5
						on table >2 hours	5
						Medication	★
						Cytotoxics	4
						High dose steroids	
						Anti-inflammatory	

Name of Nurse Completing Assessment:		
Ward/Dept:		
Signature:		
Date:	Time:	Score:
Pressure Relieving Equipment Identified:	Code no:	

Figure 3.1 Pressure ulcer risk assessment tool (reproduced with permission from Pennine Acute Hospitals).

Range of interventions (RCN 2000; NICE 2003a, b, c)

- Skin inspection regularly, in line with individualised risk areas following a head-to-foot assessment. For neurological patients this should include the scalp, the tips of the ears, elbows, ankle joints and toes as well as the more usual risk areas such as sacrum, hips and heels.
- Use of pressure-distributing device based on collaborative clinical judgement. The pressure distribution should be continued while the patient is seated.
- The following should not be used as aids: water-filled gloves, synthetic sheepskins, genuine sheepskins and doughnut-type devices.
- Repositioning should be determined by the skin inspection, take into account other activities, and be agreed with the individual and documented.
- People with absent sensation, body neglect, cognitive or perceptual problems will need extra care to protect body parts from entrapment.
- Ensure seated periods are safe and comfortable, and mirror pressure redistribution while in bed.
- Seek advice from physiotherapist where doubt or difficulty exists, particularly in transferring patients, to avoid shearing, sliding or pushing.

The Multiple Sclerosis Trust has compiled guidelines for good management of pressure risk (MST 2000) and Chapter 10 of this book discusses the principles of good positioning and postural management in more depth. Gary (see case study in the section on How to Use this Book) has poor sitting balance and is at risk not only of falling but also of getting his arms trapped either by his own body or in the side of a chair. Mark clearly has poor balance and reduced motor ability. With his head lolling forward, he is in an unstable position and could develop sacral pressure sores. Because of his poorly controlled secretions he could develop areas of excoriation around his mouth.

Risks from altered perception and cognition

In many general settings, perceptual and cognitive deficits are loosely covered by the adjectives 'wandering' or 'confused' to describe patients who may be at risk of falling or may be a danger to themselves. The term *confusion* is vague and often used to cover the many states in which a patient is unable to think and act with normal speed, clarity and coherence, and includes confusion of sudden onset as well as the more gradual progression of dementia, and perceptual deficits that may be mistaken for confusion. Impaired cognition has also been identified as an important risk factor and should be part of any instrument that is developed to assess a person's risk of falling.

The features of confusion identified by Evans *et al.* (2001) include:

- disorientation to time, place or person;
- impaired attentiveness and concentration;
- inability to register immediate events and recall them later;
- reduced perceptiveness and inappropriate interpretation of the environment;
- sometimes accompanied by visual or auditory illusions;
- sometimes stereotyped activities such as plucking at bed-clothes or 'wandering'.

Harry and Mark may well be labelled as confused, and Fred, due to his experience of visual and auditory hallucination, may also earn himself the label. However, a thorough assessment carried out by an occupational therapist can identify specific deficits for which compensatory strategies can be identified in the care plan, which can help relieve some of the manifestations such as wandering or aggression.

The specific deficits that may accompany neurological disease or injury are summarised in Table 3.7 and include the following:

- scanning deficits such that the eye cannot take in moving objects;
- loss of co-ordination of eye movements, causing double vision or inability to judge depth;
- body scheme disorder leading to poor balance and equilibrium;
- topographical disorientation with difficulty in route finding and inability to recall the spatial arrangement of familiar surroundings;

- inability to recognise familiar landmarks;
- inability to judge depth and distance (Grieve 1993).

An occupational therapy assessment, together with an assessment by a neuropsychologist or clinical psychologist, will help to determine the nature of the confusion or perceptual deficit. Compensatory strategies can be developed from this, and are discussed further in Chapter 11.

Wandering and risk

The term *wandering* is often linked with confusion. Lai and Arthur (2003) suggest that, like confusion, the term is imprecise and difficult to define. Several studies (Allan 1994; Allison and Marshall 1994; Aspinall 1994; Dewing and Blackburn 1999; Hughes 2002; Ross 2003) indicate that wandering patients present a challenge to their carers in balancing rights, risk and therapy. An effective care plan should be developed from thorough assessment and should clearly indicate a rationale for any interventions. The rationale needs to indicate in what way the interventions represent the best interests of the patient, bearing in mind the four principles of beneficence, non-maleficence, autonomy and justice (Horsburgh 2003). Most care settings have organisational policies and protocols that ensure these principles are honoured.

Nursing assessment of risk

In assessing actual and potential risk of injury or falls in restless, confused or wandering patients, nurses need to take into account the points raised in Box 3.1. It is worth noting the point made about *seizure activity*. Patients with neurological damage may well experience seizure activity that is mistaken for wandering or confusion, and there is a fuller discussion on seizure activity in Chapter 13. Many health care providers now also require nurses to complete a risk assessment for the use of bed rails and for falls, and the intervention protocols linked to assessment score (Gallinagh *et al.* 2001, 2002) Examples are shown in Figures 3.2 and 3.3. In addition, the Medical Devices Agency (2001) has produced guidelines on side rail use. Once an assessment has been made, discussions have taken place

Box 3.1 Nursing assessment of restlessness and risk

What could be causing the restlessness?

- Is it goal-directed behaviour attempting to relieve a physical discomfort such as full bladder or hunger, or emotional discomfort such as homesickness or anxiety?
- Is it a natural release for agitation, boredom or the need for social interaction?
- Is it spontaneous motor activity caused by damage to the motor cortex or motor neurones, which has not been triggered by a goal or motive?
- Is it **seizure activity**? Partial seizure activity can often be mistaken for restlessness or confusion. Patients may be wandering, fumbling, twitching or carrying out inappropriate activities because of seizure activity in the brain (Shorvon and Walker 2000).
- Is there an underlying biological cause such as infection or pain?

What are the risks to the person's well-being?

- Is there a risk of falling from weakness, spasticity, reduced perception of depth and height, reduced balance, reduced capacity to plan and execute movements or anticipate potential problems in movement?
- Are patients likely to elope? This refers specifically to patients who leave the care environment but are deemed unsafe to be alone and unsupervised in that situation because of their poor judgement of personal safety which arises from their cognitive/perceptual deficits.
- Are patients at risk of physical harm from reduced ability to interpret actual or potential dangers in the environment, such as in the kitchen, near stairs, in the bathroom or near a road? Of particular concern are potentially hazardous items such as electrical appliances, knives and feeding utensils, medications, medical equipment, household cleaning fluids, gas appliances.

The majority of falls occur at or near the patient's bed, accounting for up to 50% of falls. Other locations include corridors, bathrooms and toilets.

Risk Assessment – Use of Bed Rails

Application in accordance with the advice of July 2001 from the Medical Devices Agency. The following points are to help staff understand the need for risk assessment before bed rails are used and the specific risks associated with their use. Having taken the decision to use bed rails, staff must then complete this risk assessment form to ensure that all potential risks are considered and controlled.

Patient's name   Admission

Date of birth   Admission weight

Ward

Completion Each of the following sections must be completed by a Registered Nurse in order to be considered a suitable and sufficient assessment of risk. Should any of the conditions listed below exist then matching rails correctly fitted and in good condition must be applied to each side of the bed. Should other factors be relevant the Registered Nurse will exercise their judgement in deciding whether or not to apply rails.

Is the patient: Elderly or immobile

Suffering from cerebral palsy

Underweight or overweight

Suffering from dementia

Suffering from neurological disease

Criterion	Yes – No – N/A	If No – Further action required
1. The patient requires safety rails because ... explain		
2. The rails work correctly, are a matched pair and fit correctly on the bed.		
3. There is no perceived danger of entrapment of the patient's head, limbs, lines or drainage tubes.		
4. The patient can always be observed by staff.		
5. The patient is not under direct observation so ... describe precautions		
6. The bed will be positioned at the lowest height when staff are not at the patient's bedside.		
7. Suitable height extension rails will be used if the mattress thickness is greater than normal, or an overlay is added.		
8. Consent has been obtained from the patient/partner/next of kin. Indicate which		
Date Named nurse		

NB • This assessment must be repeated if the patient's condition changes to any significant degree.

• This assessment and any subsequent revision must be signed and dated and placed in the patient's care plan.

• File any completed assessment and subsequent revisions with the patient's notes upon discharge.

Figure 3.2 Example of risk assessment for use of bed rails.

RISK ASSESSMENT FOR FALLS

Patient Name: **Ward**

AGE / SEX	Score	BALANCE	Score	MOBILITY	Score
Under 60 yrs (0) 60–70 (1) 71–80 (2) 80+ (3) Male (1) Female (2)		Immobile/steady (0) Steady – with aid/s (1) Unsteady – declines or refuses aid/s (2) Parkinsonian gait (3)		Independent or chair bound (0) Weight bears/walks with assistance/co-operative (1) Impaired balance (2) Wandering/restless (3) Requires constant observation (4)	
MEDICATION		**PHYSICAL**		**HIP PROTECTORS**	
No meds (0) On meds but no side effects/problems (1) Slight adverse reaction to meds (2) EPSE/adverse response to meds (3) Unstable – PRN (4)		Physically fit relative to age (0) Weight loss/recent ill health (1) Marked frailty (2) Recent limb fracture or injury (3) TIAs/seizures (4)		Immobile or not required (0) Accepts help or copes well (1) Removes or refuses (2) Uncompliant or mobile and self-caring (4)	
SLEEP PATTERN		**COMPREHENSION**		**CO-OPERATION**	
Sleeps well (0) Broken sleep (1) Reversed day/night pattern (2) Minimal/no sleep (3)		Fully-aware (0) Reduced awareness but responds appropriately (1) Requires clear instructions and visual prompts (2) Receptive dysphasia/confused (3)		Fully co-operative (0) Regular reassurance and instruction (1) Verbally hostile (2) Unpredictable/variable mood (3) Physically aggressive/resistive or reluctant (4)	
CONSCIOUSNESS		**FALLS HISTORY**		**DIAGNOSIS**	
Alert (0) Reduced alertness (1) Sleepy (2) Exhausted/driven (3)		No falls known (0) Previous history (1) History and increasing frequency (2) Recent and uncontrolled (3)		Cognitively intact (0) Alzheimer's (1) Vascular (2) Lewy Body (3) Acute confusional state or unconfirmed/other (4)	

RATING SCALE		TOTAL SCORE
0–12	Low risk	
13–20	Moderate risk	
21–30	Significant risk	
30+	High risk	Date:

REVIEW DATE	SIGN

Figure 3.3 Example of risk assessment for falls (reproduced with permission from West Sussex Health and Social Care Trust).

with other members of the interdisciplinary team, and local policies and protocols have been taken into account, appropriate interventions can be selected from a range such as that listed in Box 3.2.

LEGAL AND ETHICAL ISSUES OF SAFETY AND RESTRAINT

Sometimes the care team may feel that the neurological deficit is such that some kind of restraint is necessary to prevent harm. *Restraint* can take some or all of the following forms:

Box 3.2 Possible interventions to manage risk

Environmental
- Decrease environmental clutter and obstacles and ensure bed brakes are on.
- Ensure adequate lighting.
- Nurse restless or wandering patients in a low bed. Try using cushions or a sleep system to give a sense of comfort and boundary. Position bed near nurses' station.
- Mattress by the bed to cushion any falls.
- Chairs with deep seats and appropriate back support with appropriate pressure-relieving, non-slip properties. Use safety straps or seat belts in wheelchairs.
- Use visual clues to help access to toilet, place patients near toilets and regularly offer suitable toilet facility.
- Use of alarms such as bed sensors or exit door alarms if clinically appropriate.
- Liaison with occupational therapists and physiotherapists.

Psychosocial
- Companionship, active listening, relaxation therapies, activities and programmes.
- Supervised wandering and observation.
- Continuous orientation to the environment.
- A confusion box containing items such as laundry or small objects that can be sorted and tidied.

- physical restraint of one individual by another;
- restraining equipment such as bed rails or baffle locks;
- pharmacological sedation;
- removal of equipment a patient may need to mobilise;
- electronic tagging or alarm (Hughes and Low 2002; Hughes and Campbell 2003).

Nurses need to document the nursing assessment that justifies a measure of restraint in the health care setting. Such justification may occur in the following circumstances:

- There is loss of insight that impairs the person's ability to make sound judgements about their own safety (non-maleficence). Many people with documented cognitive impairment are able to make reasonable choices about treatment options if the communication mode and style are appropriate, so this issue needs to be thoroughly assessed.
- It can be shown that an infringement of the right to autonomy and the legal right to freedom of movement is outweighed by a duty of care not to be negligent.
- It can be shown that restraint is in the best interests of the patient, taking into consideration the potential consequences of their actions if steps are not taken to protect them.

Balancing rights and risks is a complex aspect of neurological care (Hughes and Campbell 2002; Horsburgh 2003), and interventions need clear documentation, with a rationale for the therapeutic or safety rationale with regard to the patient. Most care providers now use risk assessment tools and documentation protocols to support both patients and staff in the decision-making process. Occasionally, violent or disruptive behaviour may pose a threat to staff or other patients, or uncontrolled wandering pose a severe risk to the patient's well-being. If this happens, such patients may need one-to-one supervision, possibly by a qualified mental health nurse. In addition, a neuropsychologist will need to make a specialist assessment of a challenging behaviour and recommend a management strategy or a more suitable care setting.

HARRY'S CASE

Harry (see case study in the section on How to Use this Book) is a good example of a neurological patient whose safety needs come from sensory, motor and perceptual problems, cognitive problems and seizure activity.

Sensory overload

Harry may be experiencing sensory overload. The recovery period following brain injury is often accompanied by hyper-sensitive reactions to sensory stimuli that take considerable perceptual and processing effort. This can be distressing and make a person feel agitated. Nursing actions to help can include reducing the noise in the immediate environment as far as possible, allowing only two visitors at a time (explaining to the family why), using a calm and quiet nursing approach and making sure televisions are not disturbing him. Noise from the latter may contribute to sensory overload and he may be unable to distinguish the television and reality. He may develop false beliefs about his safety, contributing to his agitation.

Restlessness, rubbing legs in bed, repetitive movements

Harry's apparent fidgeting may be due to motor restlessness, seizure activity or agitation. This motor restlessness may cause the development of friction pressure sores. At-risk areas should be protected with soft padding and he needs good nutrition to fuel the activity and maintain good skin integrity. A bed rail assessment and falls risk assessment should be carried out (see Figures 3.2 and 3.3). It is possible that the restlessness is due to seizure activity (Shorvon and Walker 2000). Nursing observation is important here and is discussed more fully in Chapter 13. If you suspect that plucking, repetitive movements or aimless wandering are caused by seizure activity, record the time and duration of activity, whether he speaks or takes any notice of his surroundings or other people, responds to his name or to touch, speaks to you or tries to push you away. Does he have any twitching, does he fumble with his clothes, or is he smacking his lips? (Chapter 13 has an example of a useful seizure activity chart.) When the activity ceases, check whether he is tired and whether he remembers anything from that period. Record all observed instances on a seizure chart as this will be used to help evaluate the efficacy of anticonvulsant medication.

Wandering and disorientation

A falls risk assessment should be carried out together with an assessment of Harry's neurological state. What are the possible causes of his wandering and disorientation? Reorientate him to his surroundings in a calm manner, be gentle and speak slowly as he may be suffering from sensory overload. He needs to trust you. Ask him specific questions gently to help him identify what it is he needs and wants. Is he a smoker and would he like to go somewhere to smoke? Does he need to go to the toilet? Is he hungry or thirsty? Give him landmarks along his route to the toilet. These could be visual, auditory or tactile. Has his memory picked up from just before he collapsed and is he trying to get home from the market? Explain where he is, what has happened, who people are, what furniture and equipment is for, where his family and friends are, when he will see them. Tell him about the care he is receiving and when certain things might happen, such as lunch or a visit. This can help develop a sense of time and clock. Keep any promises you make to him. He may like soothing music; find out what he likes to do and what his hobbies are.

Becoming abusive, demanding to go home

Other signs of agitation may include raised voice, cursing, stuttering, interrupting, high colour, clenched fists, pacing, shaking index finger and pounding the table. Most nurses find these behaviours difficult to manage in a busy, non-specialist setting. The main aim is to reduce Harry's distress by using a calming approach and trying to establish whether there are specific causes for the agitation. Speak to him quietly and gently to find out if anything particular has upset him, is worrying him or making him feel uncomfortable. Most people when angry want space rather than touch, so take a step back, standing at an angle to him rather than face on, with one foot back and knees slightly bent. Ask him to make specific behavioural changes or give specific instructions, in a quiet, firm and reassuring tone, such as,

'Sit down and discuss this'. Tell him quietly, firmly and repetitively to calm down. When his mood settles, establish rapport and listen to his real message. Has someone upset him? Is there anything that would make things better for him? Are there any complementary therapies available that might help him to feel more relaxed?

Effect on his other activities of living
A physiotherapy assessment will establish whether Harry is safe to walk to the toilet alone, either accompanied or by means of mobility aids, and an occupational therapy assessment will help to establish any cognitive or perceptual problems in route finding. If there is a shortage of staff to supervise him, or if he is unsafe to walk to the toilet alone, teach him to use a urine bottle. This can add to his sense of independence, confidence and may reduce wandering. However, he may have to be shown several times how to use it.

Sedation
It is unlikely in Harry's case that sedation would be justified. It may considerably interfere with his recovering awareness and alertness, so that if he did fall he would fall very heavily and his reactions would be slowed. Sedation can mask the underlying problem, which then remains undetected. The drowsiness may interfere with the development of a therapeutic relationship, and may make him disinclined to take enough to eat or drink, slowing the recovery and rehabilitation processes.

SUMMARY
- ❏ Good pain management depends on an assessment that identifies whether the pain is nociceptive or neuropathic.
- ❏ Nurses assess pain and the effectiveness of the pain management plan using an appropriate tool, by observation and by interpreting non-verbal clues.
- ❏ Interdisciplinary care planning ensures patients can comfortably participate in physiotherapy, occupational therapy, and speech and language therapies.
- ❏ Neurological patients have increased risk of developing pressure sores, falling or otherwise injuring themselves because

of altered sensation, altered motor ability, altered perception or cognition. The risk is also increased because of the side effects of the drugs they are prescribed.

❏ Care setting policies and protocols with regard to safe care need to be implemented to ensure patient autonomy and dignity as far as possible.

❏ Clinical judgement needs to establish the root cause and therefore relevant intervention options for patients labelled wandering or confused.

❏ The use of any form of restraint needs to be documented with a therapeutic or safety rationale.

REFERENCES

Allan, K. (1994) Dementia in acute units: wandering. *Nursing Standard* **9** (8), 32–4.

Allison, A. and Marshall, M. (1994) Dementia in acute units: the issues. *Nursing Standard* **8** (52), 28–30.

Aspinall, P. (1994) When a vulnerable patient absconds. *Journal of Clinical Nursing* **3** (2), 115–18.

Axford, J. and O'Callaghan, C. (2004) *Medicine*. Blackwell, Oxford.

Baillie, L. (1993) A review of pain assessment tools. *Nursing Standard* **7** (23), 25–9.

Bird, J. (2003) Selection of pain measurement tools. *Nursing Standard* **18** (13), 33–9.

Calne, S. M. and Kumar, A. (2003) Nursing care of patients with late stage Parkinson's disease. *Journal of Neuroscience Nursing* **35** (5), 242–51.

Carroll, D. and Bowsher, D. (1993) *Pain Management and Nursing Care*. Butterworth-Heinemann, Oxford.

Delac, K. (2002) Pain assessment in patients with cognitive impairment is possible. *Topics in Emergency Medicine* **24** (1), 52–4.

Dewing, J. and Blackburn, S. (1999) Dementia, part 4: risk management. *Professional Nurse* **14** (11), 803–5.

DoH (Department of Health) (2001) *The Essence of Care: Patient Focused Benchmarking for Health Care Practitioners*. HMSO, London.

Evans, D., Hodgkinson, B., Lambert, L. and Wood, J. (2001) Falls risk factors in a hospital setting. *International Journal of Nursing Practice* **7**, 38–45.

Feldt, K. (2000) The checklist of non-verbal pain indicators. *Pain Management Nursing* **1** (1), 13–21.

Ferrell, B. A., Ferrell, B. R. and Rivera, L. (1995) Pain in cognitively impaired nursing home patients. *Journal of Pain and Symptom Control* **10** (8), 591–8.

Flanagan, M. (1993) Pressure sore risk assessment scales. *Journal of Wound Care* **2** (3), 162–7.

Gallinagh, R., Nevin, R., Campbell, L., Mitchell, F. and Wolwick, R. (2001) Relatives' perceptions of siderail use on the older person in hospital. *British Journal of Nursing* **10** (6), 391–2.

Gallinagh, R., Nevin, R., McIroy, D., Mitchell, F., Campbell, L., Ludwick, R. and McKenna, H. (2002) The use of physical restraints as a safety measure in the care of older people in four rehabilitation wards: findings from an exploratory study. *International Journal of Nursing Studies* **39** (2).

Gray, P. and Hildebrand, K. (2000) Fall risk factors in Parkinson's disease. *Journal of Neuroscience Nursing* **32**, 222–8.

Grieve, J. (1993) *Neuropsychology for Occupational Therapists.* Blackwell Science, Oxford.

Halfens, R. J. G., Van Achterberg, T. and Bal, R. M. (2000) Validity and reliability of the Braden Scale and the influence of other risk factors: a multicentre prospective study. *International Journal of Nursing Studies* **37** (4), 313–19.

Hamilton, F. (1992) An analysis of the literature pertaining to pressure sore risk assessment scales *Journal Of Clinical Nursing* **1** (4), 185–93.

Ho, K., Spence, J. and Murphy, M. F. (1996) Review of pain measurement tools. *Annals of Emergency Medicine* **27** (4), 427–32.

Horsburgh, D. (2003) The ethical implications and legal aspects of patient restraint. *Nursing Times* **99** (6), 26–7.

Hughes, J. and Campbell, G. (2003) The electronic tagging and tracking debate. *Nursing and Residential Care* **5** (4), 174–7.

Hughes, J. C. and Low, S. J. (2002) Electronic tagging of people with dementia who wander: ethical considerations are possibly more important than practical benefits. *British Medical Journal* **325** (7369), 847–8.

Hughes, M. (2002) Best practice in fall minimization among wandering clients. *Nursing and Residential Care* **4** (11), 541–4, 550–1.

Inbody, S. B. (1998) Pain syndromes. In: Rolak, L. A. (ed.), *Neurology Secrets,* 2nd edn. Hanley & Belfus, Philadelphia.

Krulewitch, H. (2000) Assessment of pain in cognitively impaired older adults: a comparison of pain assessment tools and their use by non-professional caregivers. *Journal of the American Geriatrics Society* **48** (12), 1607–11.

Lai, C. K. Y. and Arthur, D. G. (2003) Wandering behaviour in people with dementia. *Journal of Advanced Nursing* **44** (2), 173–8.

Lawler, K. (1997) Pain assessment. *Professional Nurse Study Supplement* **13** (1), S5–S8.

Marieb, E. N. (1992) *Human Anatomy and Physiology,* 2nd edn. Benjamin Cummings, New York.

Medical Devices Agency (2001) *Advice on the Safe Use of Bed Rails,* DB 2001(04). MDA, London.

MST (Multiple Sclerosis Trust) (2000) *Multiple Sclerosis Information for Health and Social Care Professionals*. Multiple Sclerosis Trust, Letchworth.

NICE (2003a) *Multiple Sclerosis: National Clinical Guidelines for Diagnosis and Management in Primary and Secondary Care*. National Institute for Clinical Excellence/National Collaborating Centre for Chronic Conditions, London.

NICE (2003b) *Triage, Assessment, Investigation and Early Management of Head Injury in Infants, Children and Adults: Clinical Practice*. National Institute for Clinical Excellence, London, available at http://www.nice.org.uk

NICE (2003c) *Pressure Ulcer Prevention*, Clinical Guideline 7. National Institute for Clinical Excellence, London, available at http://www.nice.org.uk

RCN (Royal College of Nursing) (2000) *Risk Assessment and Prevention of Pressure Sores*. Royal College of Nursing, London.

RCP (Royal College of Physicians) (1999) *National Clinical Guidelines for Stroke*. The Intercollegiate Working Party for Stroke, National Electronic Library for Health, available at http://www.nelh.nhs.uk/guidelinesdb/html/Stroke-ft.htm

RCP (Royal College of Physicians) (2002) *National Clinical Guidelines for Stroke: Update 2002*. The Intercollegiate Working Party for Stroke, Royal College of Physicians, London.

Ricci, M. and Barker, E. (1994) Pain and headache. In: Barker, E. (ed.), *Neuroscience Nursing*. Mosby, Philadelphia.

Ross, C. (2003) Wandering or walking: understanding individual cases. *Nursing and Residential Care* **5** (6), 291–3.

Rycroft-Malone, J. (2000a) Pressure ulcer risk assessment and prevention: new guidelines for practice. *Primary Health Care* **10** (9), 32–3.

Rycroft-Malone, J. and McInness, E. (2000b) *Pressure Ulcer Risk Assessment and Prevention: Technical Report*. RCN, London.

Shorvon, S. and Walker, M. (2000) *MIMS Guide to Epilepsy*, 2nd edn. Glaxo Wellcome, Uxbridge.

Wall, D. M. and Melzack, R. (1999) *Textbook of Pain*, 4th edn. Churchill Livingstone, Edinburgh.

Wall, J. (2000) Preventing pressure sores among wheelchair users. *Professional Nurse* **15** (5), 321–4.

Waters, N. and Anderson, I. (2003) Wound care: predicting pressure ulcer risk. *Nursing Times* **99** (13), 63–5.

Widor, M., Samuelsson, L., Karlsson-Tivenius, S. and Ahlstrom, G. (2002) Long-term pain conditions after stroke. *Journal of Rehabilitaiton Medicine* **34** (4), 165–70.

Wilson, M. (2002) Overcoming the challenges of neuropathic pain. *Nursing Standard* **16** (33), 47–53.

4 Communicating

INTRODUCTION

Neurological damage nearly always affects a person's communication, even if only in very subtle ways. Despite the fact that we think of communication as verbal, non-verbal communication has been thought to account for as much as 93% of human interaction. Body language such as facial expression, eye contact, vocal tone, pace and pitch, gesture and body posture convey attitude and emotion which we process much more speedily than language (Buck 1984). Neurological damage can interfere with normal communication at this very subtle level. For example, a person with Parkinson's disease has limited facial expressiveness (Calne and Kumar 2003), and this can make interpersonal interaction and relationships difficult. Damage to cranial nerves from a stroke or motor neurone disease can cause a whispery voice, flattened tone and difficulty with articulation. Motor nerve impairment may also limit gesture and posture. The aim of this chapter is to draw attention to subtle aspects of human communication, the impairments that neurological patients may have and what interventions can reduce the impact on social interaction.

LEARNING OUTCOMES

❏ Appreciate the importance of verbal and subtle non-verbal aspects of communication.
❏ Describe and differentiate between the terms receptive dysphasia, expressive dysphasia and dysarthria.
❏ Discuss the principles of nursing assessment and management of people with communication difficulties of neurological origin.
❏ Describe the role of the speech and language therapist.

SPEECH, LANGUAGE AND PHONATION

Language is a set of symbols that a person learns to interpret and use through perception and understanding of the rules about how the symbols are used. Language consists of:

- the meaning of words (semantics);
- the sound of words (phonology);
- the rules of grammar (syntax).

Although there are many human languages, all rely on an interaction of motor, sensory, perceptual and cognitive skills to interact successfully with people, as shown in Figure 4.1. Thus, to use language effectively involves:

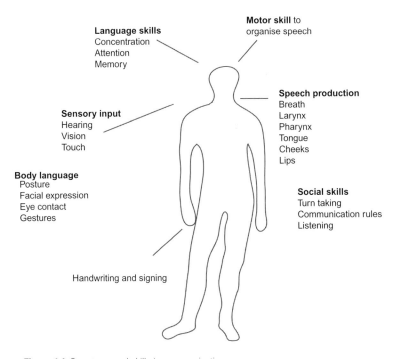

Figure 4.1 Structures and skills in communicating.

- intact sensation, particularly hearing and sight;
- accurate perception and intact cognition to interpret the sensory input;
- unimpaired motor output through the muscles of speech or writing by hand;
- impact through *voice pitch and tone* and breath control;
- control of the muscles of the throat, cheeks, tongue and lips;
- *phonation*, which refers to the sound produced from the larynx (Rolak 1998).

Before we can speak, air from the lungs has to pass through the larynx (Adam's apple). The vocal folds in the larynx vary in tension, elasticity, height, width, length and thickness because of the air passing through and the interaction of the complex sets of muscles controlling laryngeal movement. The production of sound through audible vibration of the vocal cords produces *voice or phonation*. The frequency of vibration gives us voice *quality, pitch and intonation*. Neurological conditions can often distort the normal production of speech because of damaged motor nerves to the muscles of the throat, face and mouth (see Table 4.1).

Irene (see case study in the section on How to Use this Book) has reduced voice projection and audibility because the motor neurones affecting her lung expansion and recoil are compromised. There is a reduced airflow through the vocal cords, and probably reduced function of the muscles of speech, leading to early fatigue.

Intonation means the different levels of pitch or tone used in particular sequences to express a wide range of meaning. In asking a question there is a rising pitch at the end of the question. For example the utterance 'They *are* coming here' is a declaration, while, 'They are coming *here*?', with a rise at the end, indicates a question. These words can also convey anger, surprise, sarcasm or delight by other features such as emphasis, loudness, tone of voice and facial expression. People who suffer from Parkinson's disease, motor neurone disease, or have damaged cranial nerves may have very limited ability to alter their tone or facial expression, which, when taken in conjunction with poor articulation, can make normal interaction difficult.

Table 4.1 Neurological disorders and potential communication problems.

	Altered sensation	Altered motor ability	Altered perception	Altered cognition	Communication activity
Stroke	Impaired vision Hemianopia Depression and emotionalism	Weakened cranial nerves of speech Dysarthria Articulation problems Right side weakness, asymmetrical facial expression Impaired writing ability	Depth/ foreground Visual agnosia Inability to intepret gesture	Number and letter recognition Aphasia Slowed information processing	**Fluent aphasia** (Wernicke's): good articulation and phonation, and intonation but words do not make sense **Non-fluent aphasia** (Broca's): slow laborious, halting telegrammatic Stammering
Multiple sclerosis	Blurred vision Depression	Weak muscles of throat and neck causing dysarthria, unco-ordinated arm and hand movements, impaired pen control	Visual spatial perception	Reduced attention, concentration, memory loss, and processing speed	
Parkinson's disease		Weak muscles causing voice and articulation problems, lack of facial expressiveness Small handwriting		May or may not have some dementia depending on severity	Uncontrolled saliva; some pronunciation difficulty; nasal quality; whispery, monotonous stammering, slow, slurred and indistinct

Table 4.1 *Continued*

	Altered sensation	Altered motor ability	Altered perception	Altered cognition	Communication activity
Brain injury	Possible visual, auditory impairment	Spasticity or contracture of handwriting arm, dysarthria, altered facial expressiveness Fatigue	Depth/foreground perception Visual agnosia	Number and letter recognition Aphasia Slowed information processing	Varies considerably. May lose normal social skills of interaction such as turn taking, social space and inhibition
Epilepsy	Drug therapy may cause dizziness	Drug therapy may cause fatigue, drowsiness or sedation	Drug therapy may cause double vision	Not usually affected. Partial seizures may affect concentration and memory Drug therapy may affect cognition	May be affected by slowed thought processes or memory problems
Dementia	Hearing loss Visual problems	Muscle weakness or spasticity Contractures may have developed	Visuo-spatial problems	Memory, concentration and attention problems Impaired language ability Aphasia	Word-finding problems, difficulty retaining thread of conversation
Motor neurone disease		Weak muscles of tongue and lips, soft palate, vocal cords, chest			Uncontrolled saliva; some pronunciation difficulty; nasal quality; hoarse, low-pitched, monotonous, slow, slurred and indistinct

The functions of intonation are to:

- convey emotion and attitude, e.g. friendliness, surprise, sadness, irritation;
- affect meaning, e.g. question or statement;
- emphasise words to make some words more important or prominent;
- maintain listeners' interest in lengthy utterances.

People with Parkinson's disease, such as Fred (see case study in the section on How to Use this Book), may lack much facial expression and variable voice tone. Carers would need to learn to tune into subtle alterations to pick up on his meaning.

Articulation occurs when the sound and pitch of the tone emerging from the larynx are converted by movements of the tongue, soft palate and lips to speech. The parts involved in the articulation of sound are the following:

- *Pharynx*, which is a muscular tube leading from the larynx to the back of the mouth. It can be narrowed or widened to affect sound.
- *Soft palate*, which is a broad band of muscular tissue at the back of the mouth at the top. It can be raised and lowered to help shape sound.
- *Lips*, which may be open, closed or shaped to form different sounds.
- *Jaw*, which controls the size of the gap between the upper and lower teeth and influences the position of the lips.
- *Tongue*, which is crucial to the formation of a large number of speech sounds and capable of adopting more shapes and positions than any other speech organ.

Fluency is the term used to describe smooth, rapid, effortless use of language. Fluency disorders are most noticeable when people have difficulty with the timing or rhythm of speech, as in stuttering or stammering, word-finding problems or dysarthria.

Articulation problems: dysarthria

Articulation difficulty is common in several neurological diseases such as Parkinson's disease, motor neurone disease and multiple sclerosis (see Table 4.1). In these conditions, the nerves

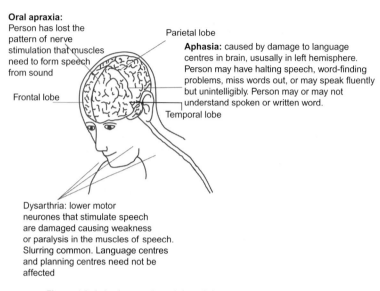

Oral apraxia:
Person has lost the pattern of nerve stimulation that muscles need to form speech from sound

Frontal lobe

Parietal lobe

Aphasia: caused by damage to language centres in brain, ususally in left hemisphere. Person may have halting speech, word-finding problems, miss words out, or may speak fluently but unintelligibly. Person may or may not understand spoken or written word.

Temporal lobe

Dysarthria: lower motor neurones that stimulate speech are damaged causing weakness or paralysis in the muscles of speech. Slurring common. Language centres and planning centres need not be affected

Figure 4.2 Aphasia, apraxia and dysarthria.

that supply the muscles are impaired. This causes indistinct speech, or dysarthria, and the problem here is one of muscle weakness and articulation not one of language processing in the brain itself (see Figure 4.2). The difficulty can make speaking very tiring and effortful. Joyce (see case study in the section on How to Use this Book) has a severe dysarthria, which makes her speech very nasal, lacking in tone with unclear articulation. This can lead to inappropriate responses from carers who may make unwarranted assumptions about cognitive damage.

There is another articulation problem known as *oral apraxia*. This means the loss of the ability to carry out skilled movements, and although not technically a language-processing problem, it causes loss of the ability to co-ordinate tongue, cheek and lip movements to produce speech. While it is not a language-processing problem, it can often follow an insult to the brain that does affect language processing, such as stroke or brain injury (Echavarri Perez 2000).

LANGUAGE CENTRES IN THE BRAIN AND APHASIA

Each hemisphere of the brain not only controls movement and sensation on the opposite side of the body but also specialises in mental functions. In most people, the left hemisphere deals with language. Neurones that produce language are clustered in an area of the left temporo-parietal lobe called Broca's area, and sensory reception of the spoken word in Wernicke's area. When these areas are damaged by a stroke, brain injury, tumour or cerebral bleed, language problems arise called aphasia or dysphasia. *Aphasia*, or *dysphasia*, means impaired ability in language, and the main types of aphasia are summarised in Table 4.2. Other impairments that may affect communication ability are summarised in Table 4.1.

ASSESSMENT AND COLLABORATIVE CARE PLANNING

Most general nursing assessment of communication is largely unstructured and develops informally while the patient is being cared for (Hemsley *et al.* 2001; Aveyard 2003). Patients and nurses develop a shared understanding using different means of communication (Sundin *et al.* 2000; Sundin and Jansson 2003). However, several studies (Reedy 1986; Bowles *et al.* 2001; Chant *et al.* 2002) show that many nurses lack the skills to assess a person's abilities and disabilities, and that as a result are not able to intervene in a way that is specific to the person's needs. There is a professional obligation in terms of informed consent (Cable *et al.* 2003), and aphasic patients present a unique group, particularly since the impairment can result in muddling head nods and head shaking.

A structured communication assessment tool may be useful, but the data that nurses gather as part of their relational rather than mechanistic communication can form an important part of the assessment and care planning when properly documented (Le Dorze *et al.* 1994; Chant *et al.* 2002)

Table 4.2 The main types of aphasia.

Type of aphasia	Location of lesion	Causes	Signs
Global	Parietal or temporo-parietal lobe, involving Broca's area and Wernicke's area	Infarction, haemorrhage, tumour	Both receptive and expressive language functions are lost. There is poor fluency, poor comprehension, poor repetition, patient may be drowsy, inattentive or apathetic. Eyes, however, may express interest or other emotional state
Broca's (motor, non-fluent, expressive aphasia	Language area of frontal lobe, usually left hemisphere	Embolism or infarction of middle cerebral artery. Possibly haemorrhage, trauma, inflammation or tumour in this anatomic region	Non-fluency (may miss words out), effort to initiate speech, poor ability to name, word-finding difficulty, fairly good comprehension. Often associated with right hemiparesis
Wernicke's (sensory, fluent, receptive aphasia)	Front of temporo-parietal lobe	Occlusion of lower division of left middle cerebral artery	Inability to understand spoken or written word, articulates spontaneously and well but uses words inappropriately, invents words, cannot repeat words. Intonation good and appropriate
Anomic	Parietal, sub-cortical or temporal lobe	Early Alzheimer's disease, metabolic confusion states, residual after recovery from Wernicke's	Can immediately repeat a spoken word, fluent output, good comprehension but lost ability to name objects, although can describe an object's colour, size, purpose

NURSING ASSESSMENT

The aims of a nursing assessment are twofold:

- *To build a trusting relationship.* The patient is then more relaxed in interaction and the lowered anxiety levels improve function. Speech and language therapists may well supplement the findings of their structured tests by discussion with relatives and nurses about communication ability in a normal social context (Schuell 1975).

- *To identify positive communication attributes* and use them to enhance the person's ability to communicate informed consent. As nurses get to know patients they respond to a patient's spontaneous compensations for communication impairment such as head nods, blinks, eyebrow flare and arch, wink, thumbs up, finger signals, facial expression, tone and pitch of sounds emitted (MacIsaac 1993). This can supplement the speech and language assessment and contribute significantly to effective care planning (Bryan 2004; Morris 2004), and should be documented in the care plan for nurses who know the patient less well.

If a structured assessment tool is used it should include hearing, vision and muscle strength (Reedy 1986) and look at specific aspects of verbal and non-verbal communication such as the following:

- *Comprehension of spoken language.* See if the person can obey simple commands such as 'Point to the chair'; then move to more complex structures using complex verbal commands for example 'Count to three then stand up using the grab rail', simple written commands, 'Open your mouth', and complex written commands, 'Open the wardrobe door, select your clothes, then close the wardrobe door'.

- *Comprehension of gestures and body language* such as head shaking, nodding, shoulder shrug, facial expressions, beckoning, hand gestures.

- *Expression in spoken language.* Word-finding ability can be assessed by asking the patient, 'Tell me the name of three things in the room'. The speech can then be assessed for fluency, speed, hesitancy, and for attempt to correct errors, and whether words are invented or circumlocution is used.

- *Expression in written language*, such as name, words, phrases or sentences, recognition of letters of simple words.
- *Ability to get message across using non-verbal gesture* (bearing in mind that paralysis or movement problems may affect this.) Head nodding, gestures, body language, sound and intonation.
- *Ability to interact* through attending to interaction, maintaining eye contact, posture, whether they stay with the topic, whether they initiate topics, can initiate interaction spontaneously and whether turn taking is understood.
- *Use of compensatory strategies.* These include use of simple speech, expanding or elaborating a message with gesture, intonation or speed, using placeholders such as 'um', 'er' and pauses, and ability in self-correcting.
- *Expression of emotions.* Conveys anger, sadness, fear, enjoyment, love, embarrassment, frustration.

Although these features may not be formally documented as part of the nursing assessment of communicative ability, Aveyard (2003) describes how nurses rely on many non-verbal features to help them grapple with the difficult issue of informed consent to care for patients who are aphasic or cognitively impaired.

The goals of therapeutic interventions are that the person is able to use a range of techniques and strategies to communicate, that the person is able to engage in meaningful interpersonal and social interaction, and that therapy programmes facilitate maximum possible recovery of language function.

ROLE OF SPEECH AND LANGUAGE THERAPIST

The nursing assessment needs also to take into account an assessment by speech and language therapists and occupational therapists, who use a range of structured assessment techniques that elicit language ability, non-verbal competence, perceptual and cognitive activity (Penn 1986; Robey 1994; Hemsley *et al.* 2001). These assessment tools help to make a systematic analysis of linguistic, perceptual and motor abilities and impairments from which to design a treatment programme. According to Greener *et al.* (2004), a speech and language therapist performs the following tasks:

- maps patterns of difficulties and recommends treatment programme activities (Byng and Black 1995);
- recognises areas of preserved ability and how to use compensatory strategies such as cueing and using alternative forms of communication such as drawing (Chapey 1986; Mitchum 1994; Hemsley *et al.* 2001);
- reduces communication stress on carers, family and friends;
- monitors and reviews difficulties and abilities over time (Kagan 1995);
- educates and trains staff, patients, family and friends in communication-related skills and provides a resource for students of several different disciplines (Le Dorze *et al.* 1994; Kagan 1995; Hemsley *et al.* 2001; Kagan *et al.* 2001);
- may be able to help in matters of advocacy and power of attorney;
- promotes good practice to achieve effective communication with people who have communication difficulties, including attention deficits (Murray 2002).

All of the patients in the case studies (see the section on How to Use this Book) will need an assessment of their communication needs, and in doing so nurses can make use of many of the tactics suggested in Box 4.1 to ensure that assessment findings are as valid as possible. The effectiveness of assessment interventions and the role of the nurse varies in different care settings (Loughrey 1992; LaBreche 1993). While nurses are involved at different levels in aphasia therapy, professional issues of informed consent and patient well-being indicate that nurses need to have their own well-developed and well-documented communicative strategies with patients (Aveyard 2003; Hayashi and Oppenheimer 2003). Several studies (Goleman 1986; BBSF 1998; Kerr and Lacelle 2000; Hilari and Byng 2001) use patient self-reports to indicate the importance of skilled communication techniques in their sense of well-being. Good collaboration among nurse, patient, speech and language therapist and the care team is thus significant in the

Box 4.1 Techniques to facilitate communication (Quigley 1992; BBSF 1998; Pound *et al.* 2000)

- Exclude competition for your attention by drawing curtains or closing doors.
- Ensure that you have the person's attention by saying their name, touching shoulder, and that they have any helpful devices to hand, e.g. spectacles, hearing aids, electronic devices, pen and paper.
- Ensure that the person is in a suitable position to make eye contact and see you. People with poor head control may need support to maintain eye contact and to see the expression on other people's faces.
- Be free with your use of facial expression and make sure the person can see your face and that you have their attention.
- Show that you feel you are talking to an intelligent person who can use their remaining capacities and skills to overcome the speaking and writing difficulty.
- Speak clearly and simply, form your words fully but do not speak too loudly and not as though you were talking to a child. Use the assessment findings to construct verbal interaction to the person's abilities. Break up sentences to make one point at a time, try rephrasing if the person has not understood. Do not change topic too quickly.
- Remember that although the person may not respond immediately, they may be processing your communication or planning how to respond. Remember to give people time, particularly since many neurological patients have slowed processing ability.
- Use humour to lighten the situation if that is appropriate.
- Take note of the gestures people use (thumbs up, or holding one finger up), their facial expressions (eyebrow raising, winking, screwing up face), and the other compensatory strategies they may be using. Establish reliability of head nodding and shaking, especially in patients

who have had a stroke. Include this in care plan documentation.

- Respond to any signals that show that they have understood by checking your understanding of the signal/sign with them. Discuss with other staff and document the ability.
- Use partners, relatives, friends who have an intimate knowledge of the person's body language and facial expressions and communication style. Encourage relatives and friends to bring in photographs and familiar items.
- Use all possible means of communicating at your disposal. Write things down, point to pictures (using a communication board), use exaggerated gestures and mime, touch if appropriate, electronic devices, picture boards, letterboards, magic slates, pen and paper.
- Remember that people may gain a lot of meaning from the context in which they see the nurse speaking.
- Remember that patients will pick up non-verbal information about you, your mood and your attitude.

Techniques for communicating with people with dysarthria

- Patients with dysarthria may not have any comprehension difficulty and it may not be necessary to slow down your speech, alter your vocabulary or sentence structure.
- Give people plenty of time to form their words, remembering that the words at the end of a sentence may be more indistinct as they fatigue. Show what you have understood and only ask them to repeat indistinct words.
- Remind people to use their communication aids if they tire.
- Ask them to spell or give the first letter of a word that you have not understood, and guess to see if you are right.

success of a person's recovery of language, effectiveness of compensatory strategies and sense of well-being (Blomert 1995).

OTHER COMMUNICATION PROBLEMS AND OCCUPATIONAL THERAPY

Some neurological conditions involve other perceptual and cognitive problems (Goldberg 1998; Wilson 1999) that can affect communication and interpersonal skills (see Table 4.1). Therapy devised by occupational therapists is aimed at redeveloping skills in focusing attention, retraining memory, teaching compensation approaches, practising perceptual ability through activities such as object and symbol recognition. These aspects are dealt with in Chapter 11. If an integrated care plan is developed by the team, it draws attention to the opportunities nurses have in their interactions with patients to help them use compensatory strategies in everyday activity, conversation and interaction. For example, brain injury may leave a person with altered social skills and lack of inhibition. Patients become less adept at the social aspects of communication such as turn taking, maintaining personal space and using acceptable vocabulary skills (Cheung and Broman 1999). Nurses, because of their natural interaction with patients and their families in everyday activities, can easily help patients to redevelop social skills. Harry's behaviour, for example, presents socially unacceptable communications, and modification of this behaviour is an important part of helping him relearn social skill and appropriateness.

ELLA'S CASE

Ella's stroke has affected her speech. She may be emotional and upset because of this and because of disturbances within her brain. Her nurse should explain all interventions and procedures carried out, involving Ella to negotiate consent, and she may need to use pointing and gesture. Very often patients not only have expressive problems but also have receptive disturbances which may take the form of not being able to understand the spoken word or having difficulty recognising familiar objects. The nurse should refer her to an occupational therapist when she is over the very acute stage, whose assessment will identify any perceptual deficits. The nurse should also refer Ella to speech and language therapy for a communication assessment (RCP 1999). That assessment will provide treatment and strategy recommendations that will help Ella to identify everyday objects that she may need. She could be provided with a pencil and paper as she may find it easier to write things down. In addition, those nursing Ella should allow her time to answer any questions and should keep sentences short and uncomplicated. She is a young woman who has worked in a medical environment for a number of years. This needs to be taken into account, as she may need fuller explanations about what has happened to her than do other patients who do not have a similar background.

JOYCE'S CASE
Joyce has difficulty in articulation, and her speech may be slurred or drunken sounding. Her rate of speech may be slow, unmelodic and flattened in tone. Nurses need to encourage Joyce to maintain a good posture while she speaks, get her to take appropriate breaths and to break up words if necessary, and give her time. In addition, her nurses need the skills to phrase questions in such a way that Joyce can give short answers.

Compensatory strategies may include supplying Joyce with assistive devices such as a pen and paper, communication board or light writer.

SUMMARY
❏ Neurological disturbance may cause problems with speech production (dysarthria) or language processing (aphasia or dysphasia) or other impairments that may reduce social skill and normal inhibition.
❏ The effectiveness and impact of verbal communication is strongly influenced by accompanying features such as phonation, intonation, articulation, facial expression and gesture.
❏ Nursing assessment involves a range of verbal and non-verbal features (in structured and unstructured ways) of a patient's communication attempts in order to plan effective

goals and interventions and to give a rationale for consent being given.

❏ Nursing skills take into account the environment, the kinds of impairments that are causing communication difficulty, and the use of a range of techniques to facilitate communication.

❏ Communication needs to include planned and paced inter-actions, and involve liaison with family, speech and language therapists and occupational therapists.

❏ Communication can be enhanced with the use of simple devices such as pen or paper, sign language, communication boards or electronic equipment recommended by speech and language therapists.

❏ The process of communicating with aphasic patients raises difficult issues of informed consent.

REFERENCES

Aveyard, H. (2003) The patient who is unable to consent to nursing care. *International Journal of Nursing Studies* **40**, 697–705.

BBSF (British Brain and Spine Foundation) (1998) *Speech, Language and Communication Difficulties.* BBSF, London.

Blomert, L. (1995) Who's the expert? Amateur and professional judgment of aphasic communication. *Topics in Stroke Rehabilitation* **2** (3), 64–71.

Bowles, N., Mackintosh, C. and Torn, A. (2001) Nurses communi-cation skills: an evaluation of the impact of solution focused com-munication training. *Journal of Advanced Nursing* **36** (3), 347–54.

Bryan, K. (2004) *What Can Speech and Language Therapy Offer in the Early Stages of Dementia.* Mental Health Foundation, available at http://www.mhilli.org/network/speechlanguage.htm

Buck, R. (1984) *The Communication of Emotion.* Guilford Press, New York.

Byng, S. and Black, M. (1995) What makes a therapy? Some para-meters of therapeutic intervention in aphasia. *European Journal of Disorders of Communication* **30**, 303–16.

Cable, S., Lumsdaine, J. and Semple, M. (2003) Informed consent. *Nursing Standard* **18** (12), 47–53.

Calne, S. M. and Kumar, A. (2003) Nursing care of patients with late stage Parkinson's disease. *Journal of Neuroscience Nursing* **35** (5), 242–51.

Chant, S., Jenkinson, T., Randle, J., and Russell, G. (2002) Commu-nication skills: some problems in nursing education and practice. *Journal of Clinical Nursing*, **11** (1), 12–21.

Chapey, R. (1986) Language intervention strategies adult aphasia. In Florrence, C. L. and Conway, W. F. (eds) *Transdisciplinary Intervention*. Williams & Williams, New York.

Cheung, M. E. and Broman, S. H. (1999) Adaptive learning: interventions for verbal and motor deficits. *Neurorehabilitation and Neural Repair* **14** (3), 159–69.

Echavarri Perez, C. (2000) Communication and language impairments in cerebral injury. *Rehabilitation* **34** (6), 483–91.

Goldberg, G. (1998) What happens after brain injury? You may be surprised at how rehabilitation can help your patient. Symposium: second of four articles on care after neurological injury. *Postgraduate Medicine* **104** (2), 91–4, 99–105, 175–7.

Goleman, D. (1996) *Emotional Intelligence*. Bloomsbury, London.

Greener, J., Enderby, P. and Whurr, R. (2004) Speech and language therapy for aphasia following stroke. The Cochrane Library, Oxford.

Hayashi, H. and Oppenheimer, E. A. (2003) ALS patients on TPPV: totally locked in state, neurologic findings and ethical implications. *Neurology* **61** (1), 135–7.

Hemsley, B., Sigafoss, J., Balandin, S., Forbes, R., Taylor, C., Green, V. A. and Parmenter, T. (2001) Nursing the patient with severe communication impairment. *Journal of Advanced Nursing* **35** (6), 827–35.

Hilari, K. and Byng, S. (2001) Measuring quality of life in people with aphasia: the Stroke Specific Qualtiy of Life Scale. *International Journal of Language and Communication Disorders* **36** (Supplement), 86–91.

Kagan, A. (1995) Revealing the competence of aphasic adults through conversation: a challenge to health professionals. *Topics in Stroke Rehabilitation* **2** (1), 15–28.

Kagan, A., Black, S. E. Duchan, J. F. Simmons-Mackies, N. and Square, P. (2001) Training volunteers as conversation partners using 'Supported Conversation for Adults with Aphasia' (SCA): a controlled trial. *Journal of Speech, Language and Hearing Research* **44** (3), 624–38.

Kerr, N. and Lacelle, B. (2000) Therapy for aphasia: insiders points of view . . . including commentary by Elman R. J. *Journal of Medical Speech – Language Pathology* **8** (2), 103–31.

Labreche, J. (1993) Rehabilitation nurses and speech therapy. *Rehabilitation Nursing* **18** (1), 54.

Le Dorze, G., Julien, M., Brassard C., Durochet, J. and Bolvin, G. (1994) An analysis of the communication of adult residents of a long term care hospital as perceived by their caregivers. *European Journal of Disorders of Communication* **29**, 241–67.

Loughrey, L. (1992) The effects of two teaching techniques on recognition and use of function words by aphasic stroke patients. *Rehabilitation Nursing* **17** (3), 135–7.

MacIsaac, E. (1993) Answer that soon. *Nursing Times* **89** (1), 43.

Mitchum, C. (1994) Traditional and contemporary views of aphasia: implications for clinical management. *Topics in Stroke Rehabilitation* **1** (2), 14–36.

Morris, C. (2004) *Communication Problems in Dementia*, Pick's Disease Support Group Factsheet, available at http://www.pdsg.org.uk/Factsheets/communication.htm.

Murray, L. L. (2002) Attention deficits in aphasia: presence, nature, assessment, treatment *Seminars in Speech and Language* **23** (2), 107–16.

Penn, C. (1986) Compensation and language recovery in chronic aphasia. *British Journal of Disorders in Communication* **21**, 239–45.

Pound, C., Parr, S., Lindsay, J. and Woolf, C. (2000) *Beyond Aphasia: Therapies for Living with Communication Disabilities*. Winslow Press, Bicester.

Quigley, P. A. (1992) Effectiveness of selected nursing interventions on the conservation of aphasic patients' energy and integrity. Unpublished PhD thesis, University of Florida.

RCP (Royal College of Physicians) (1999) *National Clinical Guidelines for Stroke*. Royal College of Physicians, London.

Reedy, D. F. (1986) The client with aphasia. *Topics in Clinical Nursing* **8** (1), 67–73.

Robey, R. R. (1994) The efficacy of treatment for aphasic persons: a meta-analysis. *Brain and Language* **47**, 582–608.

Rolak, L. A. (1998) *Neurology Secrets*, 2nd edn. Hanley & Belfus, Philadelphia.

Schuell, H. (1975) *Aphasia in Adults*. Harper & Row, New York.

Sundin, K., Jansson, L. and Norberg, A. (2000) Communicating with people with stroke and aphasia: understanding through sensation without words. *Journal of Clinical Nursing* **9**, 481–8.

Sundin, K. and Jansson, L. (2003) 'Understanding and being understood' as a creative caring phenomenon – in care of patients with stroke and aphasia. *Journal of Clinical Nursing* **12**, 107–16.

Wilson, B. (1999) *Cognitive Problems Following Stroke*. The Stroke Association, London.

Breathing

5

INTRODUCTION

All of human activities use up oxygen, which is supplied through effective breathing, good ventilation and efficient clearance of secretions. The concentrations of oxygen and carbon dioxide in the body help regulate breathing, ensure efficient cell metabolism and maintain homeostasis. The normal breathing patterns and clearance of secretions can be compromised in patients with several different neurological conditions. Brain injury or insult that causes swelling and raised intracranial pressure can impede the respiratory centre in the brain stem and cause respiratory abnormalities or arrest. The cranial and spinal nerves can be damaged by injury, and by motor neurone disease, multiple sclerosis and Parkinson's disease. Several motor nerves innervate the muscles of respiration in the head, neck, lungs and diaphragm, and damage can cause poor airflow, air control and ventilation. This creates a potential for the retention of carbon dioxide leading to acidosis, inadequate ventilation and hypoxaemia, which may in turn lead to confusion and cardiac arrhythmias. The resulting weakness in respiratory muscles creates the potential for the development of a chest infection if the secretions and contents of the alimentary tract find their way into the airway system. The problems that neurological patients experience may be sudden, acute and life threatening, as in brain injury or more insidious such as in Guillain-Barré, multiple sclerosis or motor neurone disease. These homeostatic problems render patients vulnerable to chest infection and limit their activities because of low circulating oxygen levels. The aims of this chapter are to describe the physiological background to breathing problems of neural origin and to raise awareness of a core skill set in monitoring respiratory function and preventing complications and discomforts.

LEARNING OUTCOMES
❏ Explain the role of the central nervous system and peripheral nervous system in maintaining a clear airway and in regulating respiration.
❏ Describe how to maintain the airway of a patient with neurological impairment and prevent chest infection due to aspiration of secretions.
❏ Appreciate how suctioning, humidification and tracheostomy care affect patient physical and emotional well-being.
❏ Appreciate the role of other disciplines in helping patients to maintain a clear airway.

MECHANISMS OF RESPIRATION
Nerve control of the breathing, heart rate and blood pressure is located in the brain stem. Interactions of this tissue with the cranial and spinal nerves maintain homeostasis and respiratory problems can occur when either the brain or peripheral nerves are damaged. These may become evident as hypoxaemia, communication problems or chest infection. The vagus nerve is particularly important because it arises in the brain stem and makes contact with the lungs, heart, and gastrointestinal tract and is crucial in the control of respiratory, cardiovascular and gastrointestinal function.

Inspiration occurs when new air is drawn into the lungs. The peripheral nerves supplying the diaphragm make it flatten, which makes the lungs get bigger. This makes the air pressure inside the lungs less than outside and air enters and expands the lungs. The process of inspiration normally takes about 2 seconds.

• Inspiratory neurons are stimulated by incoming messages from the apneustic centre in the brain stem and from chemical receptors.
• Inspiratory neurones then send messages down the spinal cord, some of which leave the spinal cord at the cervical vertebrae (C3, C4 and C5), to travel along the the nerves that supply the lungs. These then stimulate the diaphragm to contract and flatten. Other nerves leave the spinal cord at the tho-

racic vertebrae (T3, T4 and T5). These travel along the intercostal nerves (part of peripheral nervous system) to stimulate intercostal muscles.

After inspiration the nerve stimulation of the diaphragm muscle ceases, the diaphragm relaxes and rises. This reduces the thoracic space and lung size. Air pressure is then greater inside the lungs than outside the lungs and air is *expired* passively. Expiration would normally take about 3 seconds. Thus one complete breath normally takes about 5 seconds, giving a normal, resting breathing rate of about 10–12 breaths per minute.

The pneumotaxic centre in the brain stem modulates the process of breathing, which is why a raised intracranial pressure is so important. In addition, the lungs are protected by the epiglottis, which is controlled by the cranial nerves and which occludes entry to the lungs during swallowing. Any patient who has weakened motor ability or spasticity in this area is at risk of aspirating secretions, food or fluid down into the lung. Irene, Miriam and Joyce (see case studies in the section on How to Use this Book) are particularly vulnerable in this respect.

Other homeostatic mechanisms also regulate the rhythm and rate:

• *Chemical regulation.* A rise in carbon dioxide levels stimulates the respiratory centres giving increased rate and depth. When the carbon dioxide level falls, shallower breathing follows.
• *Blood temperature.* An increase in blood temperature will quicken but not deepen respirations. A drop in temperature slows the respiratory rate.
• *Blood pressure.* An increase in blood pressure, detected by receptors in the aorta cause a decrease in the respiratory rate. A decrease in blood pressure increases the respiratory rate.
• *Irritation of airways.* Mechanical or chemical irritation of the airways causes breathing to cease, which may be followed by sneezing, coughing or vomiting to expel the irritant, a process mediated by the medulla. In coughing and sneezing, a short inspiration is followed by a series of forced expirations.
• *Skin.* Painful or hot or cold stimuli to the skin can trigger a reflex that increases the rate and depth of breathing.

- *Muscles.* If the proprioceptors in the intercostal, diaphragm or abdominal muscles are stimulated, spasmodic contraction of the diaphragm can occur (hiccoughs).
- *Pain and strong emotion.* Sudden pain or strong emotion can cause a brief cessation of breathing. The return of breathing is characterised by the 'gasp'. Breathing is also affected by strong emotion expressed as laughter or crying. This response is mediated by the hypothalamus sending signals down to the respiratory centres in the medulla. Anxiety may cause excessively rapid, shallow breathing and result in light-headedness or fainting.

RESPIRATORY PROBLEMS OF NEUROLOGICAL ORIGIN

Trauma, infarction or infection of the motor pathways in the brain and peripheral nerves can lead to a number of abnormal breathing patterns that may be dangerous. These can be life threatening and patients will need ventilatory support to help maintain adequate oxygenation, or intervention to correct the ensuing chest infection. Problems of neurological origin are shown in Table 5.1.

ASSESSMENT

Respiratory assessment takes into account the efficacy of breathing, the work of breathing and adequacy of ventilation (Jevon and Ewens 2002). Monitoring breathing efficacy includes an assessment of the *rate, depth and rhythm* of breathing. The normal respiratory rate is 12–18 beats per minute. An increase usually occurs in activity, exercise, when people are anxious or in pain, have a pyrexia, are in shock or have some airway obstruction. A slower breathing rate occurs in brain injury and increased intracranial pressure.

ELLA'S CASE

Ella (see case study in the section on How to Use this Book) would probably have a slowed breathing rate when first admitted to hospital because of the rise in intracranial pressure pressing down on the respiratory centre. The depth of her respiration can be estimated by watching the movements of her chest wall.

Table 5.1 Breathing problems of neurological origin.

	Altered sensation	Altered motor ability	Altered perception and cognition	Breathing activity
Stroke / acquired brain injury	May lose sensation of food and fluid in the mouth	Swallowing problems		At risk of aspiration pneumonia, airway occlusion from obstruction by the tongue, from ineffective airway clearance, or silent aspiration of secretions, fluids or food
Guillain-Barré		Inflammation of nerves makes muscles of respiration weak		Patients may need ventilation through a tracheostomy tube
Multiple sclerosis		May have weakened cough reflex, reduced ability to control saliva secretions		Risk of developing chest infection May fatigue easily
Motor neurone disease		May affect motor neurones supplying muscles of throat, lungs and diaphragm		Problems with coughing, co-ordinating muscles of breathing and swallowing, reduced breathing depth and rate
Spinal damage		Diaphragm may be paralysed Intercostal muscles weakened Impaired nerve supply to abdominal muscles		High risk of developing respiratory problems
Low awareness/ Persistent vegetative state	Sensory impairment of presence of secretions	Cough reflex may be impaired Immobile and at risk of hypostatic pneumonia		High risk of developing chest infection
Dementia/global brain damage			May be unable to distinguish edible from inedible substances and objects	May be at risk of choking

In addition, she may show involvement of her accessory muscles of breathing in the neck and abdomen or nasal flaring that can indicate a breathing difficulty. A peak flow meter will give a more objective measurement of the depth of respirations. Listening to the sounds of her breathing, as indicated below, will also give an indication of the nature of any abnormalities, and pulse oximetry will give an indication of oxygen saturation of the blood, as will her skin colour such as pallor.

Abnormal breath sounds, rattling, wheezing or shortness of breath may indicate a chest infection, and there may be other signs of infection such as a raised temperature. In addition, chest infection may give rise to increased confusion due to increased carbon dioxide levels and hypoxaemia. A sputum specimen should be collected, peak flow measured and an estimate of oxygen saturation levels made.

Gurgling or wet sounds indicate fluid in the upper airway because of ineffective clearance of secretions. If these are not cleared, there is an imbalance in ventilation and oxygen intake. The presence of secretions reduces this amount and perfusion, which is the blood exchange in the alveoli. The main risks of ineffective airway clearance are complete or partial obstruction of the airway or aspiration of food and fluid into the trachea and lungs, causing infection. Checks should be made on the colour, consistency and amount of secretions for signs of infection, trauma, dehydration or evidence of aspirated food or stomach contents, which may be caused by any of the factors shown in Table 5.1.

INTERVENTIONS

The main goal of nursing interventions is to facilitate airway clearance. Interventions to achieve this may include some or all of the following:

- When the patient is lying in bed, maintain alternate side lying, supported by pillows, with head of bed elevated. This should aid the movement of secretions mechanically and by gravity and may help expectoration. Keep the head of the bed elevated or maintain a side lying position after meals to minimise the potential for regurgitation and aspiration. When sitting in a chair, make sure that the position is maintained with support and that the chin is not flexed down towards the chest. For patients who have an impaired swallow, provide small, frequent meals of a suitable consistency and consider the use of an upper gastrointestinal stimulant such as metaclopramide to reduce the potential for regurgitation.

- Provide oral hygiene after meals to prevent aspiration of food particles.
- Assess the need for suctioning, identifying how frequently oral secretions need to be assessed and managed, anticipating the need for an artificial airway if secretions cannot be cleared. The decision to use suction needs to be supported by clear clinical reasoning (Place and Fell 1998; Wainwright and Gould 1996) based on the following criteria:

  - If secretions are visible or audible or the patient complains of feeling secretions on the chest, the best option is to create the conditions where the patient has the best chance of clearing these independently by coughing or positioning. Changing the position of the patient from one side to the other with head, neck and chest well supported at a 45 degree angle may help loosen the secretions and trigger the cough reflex. If this is unsuccessful or the patient has no cough reflex or an ineffective cough reflex, they may develop hypoxaemia. Ineffective coughing makes patients vulnerable to chest infection. A reduction in arterial blood gas values may initially be detected by a falling pattern of oxygen saturation levels detected by pulse oximetry. This may be caused by airways partially obstructed by secretions, and may be relieved by suctioning. Pulse oximetry readings that are below SpO_2 90% are cause for concern (the normal range is 95–100%), and may occur before visible cyanosis.

- The aim of suctioning is to remove secretions with a minimum of hypoxaemia and tissue damage. Use suction according to current guidelines and have appropriate suctioning equipment to hand (see Box 5.1).
- Thick secretions too sticky to be expelled can trigger unrelieved coughing. In this case, a saline nebuliser may help to liquefy secretions and aid natural expulsion or suction.

Box 5.1 Suctioning procedure (Moore 2003, reproduced with permission)

- Communicate with patient and obtain verbal consent (if able).
- Explain the procedure to the patient (Mallet and Dougherty 2000).
- Organise equipment and check that the suction machine is on (Mallet and Dougherty 2000).
- Set at appropriate suction pressure – between 80 and 120 mmHg (12–16 Kpa) (Luce *et al.* 1993).
- Calculate appropriate catheter size – for endotracheal and tracheostomy tubes the catheter size should not be larger than half the diameter of the tube (Wood 1998). Some patients may require hyperoxygenation and hyperinflation before suctioning.
- If possible, the patient should be sitting in an upright position.
- Wash hands.
- Use a sterile, disposable glove on the hand manipulating the catheter (Ward *et al.* 1997) and a clean, disposable glove on the other (Mallet and Dougherty 2000).
- With the clean, disposable-gloved hand, withdraw catheter from sleeve.
- Remove the oxygen supply – for ventilator-dependent patients the length of time taken from disconnection of

---

oxygen supply to reconnection should take not more than 10 seconds (Day *et al.* 2002a).

- Introduce the suction catheter gently via the selected route.
- Do not apply negative pressure on insertion.
- On withdrawing the catheter, slowly apply suction pressure by placing the thumb over the suction port control.
- Withdraw catheter gently without rotating the catheter. Multiple-eyed catheters have holes around their diameters and hence the rotating method is unnecessary.
- Reconnect oxygen supply/apparatus as soon as possible.
- Monitor oxygen saturation levels and heart rate for any decrease indicating hypoxaemia throughout the procedure.
- Wrap the catheter around gloved hand, then pull the glove back over soiled catheter and discard safely (Mallet and Dougherty 2000).
- Rinse connection by dipping its end in the jug of sterile water (Mallet and Dougherty 2000) and discard other glove.
- Wash hands with bactericidal alcohol hand rub.
- Assess the patient and if further suctioning is required start the procedure again with another sterile catheter and glove.
- Repeat until the airway is clear (auscultate chest post-suctioning). However, no more than a total of three suction passes are recommended (Glass and Grap 1995).
- The patient should be allowed to rest between each suction pass. Evaluate effectiveness by conducting a comprehensive post-suctioning respiratory assessment (Glass and Grap 1995).
- Wash hands after suctioning (Parker 1999).
- Clean the patient's oral cavity.
- Document findings, including colour, consistency and amount of secretions.
- Allow patient to rest before taking arterial blood for analysis (Hilling *et al.* 1992).

SUCTIONING

Routes of suctioning
- *Oral.* This removes secretions from the mouth using a Yankauer suction catheter.
- *Oropharyngeal.* The catheter passes through the mouth to suction secretions from the back of the throat. A Guedel airway may be needed to assist the passage of the catheter.
- *Nasopharyngeal.* The catheter passes through the nose to remove accumulation of secretions and again may need an adjuvant airway.
- *Nasotracheal.* The catheter passes through the nose and pharynx to reach secretions in the trachea.
- *Tracheal.* The catheter passes through a tracheostomy tube. The mere presence of the tube will increase secretion production.
- *Endotracheal.* The catheter passes through endotracheal tube. This technique is highly unlikely on general wards.

Hazards of suctioning
Despite the importance of suctioning, several undesirable or potentially serious effects (Moore 2003) accompany it:

- Increased intrathoracic pressure and increased intracranial pressure.
- Stimulation of vagus nerve caused by catheter touching wall of the trachea, which may cause hypotension, arrhythmias or a feeling of faintness.
- Decreases in arterial oxygenation caused by suctioning of alveolar oxygen (Taylor-Piliae 2002).
- Introduction of nosocomial infection.
- Increased bronchospasm or paroxysmal coughing caused by irritation of tracheal mucosa.
- Atelectasis (collapse of alveoli) caused by high suction pressure and drying of secretions.
- Mucosal trauma.
- Pneumothorax.

Current recommended suctioning procedure is described in Box 5.1 (Griggs 1998; Day *et al.* 2002a,b; Moore 2003). Several studies (Macmillan 1995; Blackwood 1998; Day *et al.* 2002b) indicate that technique problems persist in practice. One study (Macmillan 1995) demonstrated that there was significant disagreement among nurses working in paediatrics over catheter size, suction pressure and method of suction as well as use of pre-oxygenation and knowledge of adverse effects. Day *et al.* (2002b) showed that among nurses working in acute and high dependency ward areas there were discrepancies in recommended practice in relation to post-suctioning auscultation, pre-oxygenation, using appropriate catheter size, using excessively high suction pressures, time before reconnection of oxygen, patient reassurance, and hand washing and goggle wearing.

Post-suction monitoring and evaluation

It is recommended that a comprehensive respiratory assessment takes place following suctioning (Glass and Gap 1995). The assessment should include the following:

- breathing sounds, including auscultation;
- skin colour;
- breathing pattern and rate;
- pulse rate;
- colour, consistency and volume of secretions – close inspection of the secretions can indicate infection and can also alert nurses to the aspiration or leakage of feed;
- signs of trauma such as bleeding;
- pain and fear – patients should be allowed time to communicate their feelings before and after suctioning, and verbal communication together with reassuring touch may help with patients with low awareness (Jablonski 1994; Thompson 2000);
- pulse oximetry;
- force and effectiveness of coughing;
- blood oxygen levels in the more acutely ill patient.

TRACHEOSTOMY

A temporary opening into the trachea may need to be made in neurological emergencies such as in brain injury or may be longer term for low-awareness patients or as a palliative measure in advanced neurological disease. There are several different kinds of tracheostomy tube, made of silver, plastic or silicone, which may be plain, cuffed or fenestrated. The most commonly used tracheostomy tubes are Shiley plastic tubes (Laws-Chapman 1998; Serra 2000; Tamburri 2000; Ede and McGowan 2001; Harkin and Russell 2001; Docherty and Bench 2002).

The frequency of care depends on the amount of secretions the patient is producing and on clinical reasoning (Clarke 1995). The inner tube should be removed at least daily, more often if secretions are troublesome, and a spare one inserted. The dirty inner tube should be cleaned with sodium bicarbonate and stored dry ready for the next change (Jamieson *et al.* 2002).

The stoma dressing should also be changed at least daily using aseptic technique and the site cleansed with 0.9% normal saline. This is also a good time to check for new hair growth on the neck which may be growing under the dressing or down the stoma site. The tracheostomy tapes should be renewed at the dressing change or whenever they are damp or soiled as this causes chaffing. They should be tied to allow one finger width between the tapes and the neck (Jamieson *et al.* 2002).

Humidification

Air is normally warmed and humidified by the nose, and the presence of a tracheostomy causes cold, dry air to reach the lungs. In addition, the air partially bypasses the full cough reflex although some contents can be expelled through the tracheal opening. The secretions in the trachea and bronchi become dry and static which can lead to collapse of the alveoli, pulmonary infection, difficulty expectorating secretions and obstruction of the tracheal tube by plugs of mucus. Humidification is essential to prevent this situation from developing. There are several methods of humidification, of which nebulisation is the most effective and safe (Buglass 1999).

- *Moist gauze veils* that are held in position across the front of the tracheostomy tube by tapes held tied loosely round the neck. These are commonly known as bibs but are not favoured because of the risks of infection.

- *Tracheostomy covers* fit at the entrance to the tube. They are made of foam that retains moisture and warmth from the expired air, which then humidifies inspired air. Once more, there is a risk of infection and staff need proper training in their management.
- *Heat and moisture exchangers* are cylindrical devices attached to the tracheostomy tube that trap the warmth and moisture of expired air and transfer it across to inspired air. The disadvantages are that the patient can cough them off and that they can fill up with secretions. However, they can be useful on certain occasions: for example, if the patient is going outside, the exchanger can modify the shock of the colder outside air.
- *Saline nebulisers* provide air that is saturated by a fine mist of moisture and can be administered by a tracheostomy mask.

MANAGEMENT OF SECRETIONS

- *Thick, tenacious secretions.* There is no conclusive evidence to suggest that instillation of normal saline before suctioning increases the removal of secretions, and several disadvantages have been identified (Hagler and Traver 1994; Jablonski 1994; Blackwood 1999; Kinloch 1999; Neill 2001; Akglu and Akyolcu 2002). If tenacious secretions are a problem they can sometimes be loosened by beta-blockers or mucolytics such as mucodyne.
- *Loose secretions, excessive secretions.* While humidification helps to keep secretions loose and moist, excess secretion can be triggered by the irritation of suctioning. Certain drugs, such as hyoscine patches can be used. These patches are usually placed behind the ear and renewed every 72 hours. However, if a reaction occurs at this site they can be placed elsewhere on the body, such as on the back. If these are unsuccessful, atropine can be used.

MANAGING DROOLING

Saliva and mucus may escape from the mouth because of poor lip seal and impaired ability to swallow. This can lead to drooling and many people feel embarrassed and ashamed as a result.

Excessive watery saliva can be controlled by atropine preparations or by sublingual, nebulised, subcutaneous or patch preparations of hyoscine. In some cases a tricyclic antidepressant, such as amitriptyline has the side effect of drying the mouth. (MND Society 2004).

Other suggestions for improving saliva control include:

- altering the position to make it easier for the person to swallow;
- using a collar that supports the head in a comfortable position;
- liaising with speech and language therapist for swallowing therapy;
- oral swabbing;
- use of suction pump;
- adapt clothing to incorporate discreet waterproof-backed insert.

Mark (see case study in the section on How to Use this Book) may have damage to the cranial nerves that regulate saliva production and muscular control of the swallowing process. If his lip control and head and neck control are weak, the problem may be made worse and he will need to be positioned carefully whether he is lying down or sitting, to prevent aspiration and choking.

INTERDISCIPLINARY CARE IN MANAGING AND PREVENTING RESPIRATORY PROBLEMS

In addition to the bedside nursing assessment, assisted by measuring technologies such as pulse oximetry and peak flow measurements, the nursing care plan can be considerably enhanced by including some aspects of assessment and intervention carried out by physiotherapists, speech and language therapists and occupational therapists (Tantucci *et al.* 1994; Gosselink *et al.* 2000).

- *Physiotherapy assessment* of neurological patients with respiratory muscle weakness can ascertain the effectiveness of the cough, the condition of the diaphragm, fatigue and vital capacity. The physiotherapist can advise on breathing exercises, intermittent positive pressure breathing, assisted coughing and careful positioning, which can all help to improve breathing function.

- *Speech and language therapists* can use coloured dye assessments (Peruzzi *et al.* 2001), video fluoroscopy and fibre optic evaluation of swallowing. These can delineate the nature, extent and severity of swallowing and the risk for aspiration. They can then advise nurses of potentially helpful therapies, manoeuvres, positioning and dietary modifications that may help avoid aspiration.

- *Occupational therapy assessments* can also advise on suitable positioning and devices that assist in activities such as eating and drinking when there is a risk of aspiration (Weins *et al.* 1999).

LONG-TERM MECHANICAL VENTILATION

For some patients, for example patients with spinal nerve damage or with motor neurone disease, long-term mechanical ventilation is an option either through a tracheostomy or through non-invasive nasal or facial masks. There is growing debate on the ethical issues (Oppenheimer 1993; Kent 1996; Baker 2001; Hayashi and Oppenheimer 2003), and the social, financial and emotional implications for family and caregivers (Moss *et al.* 1993; Spence 1995). The Motor Neurone Disease Society website has useful resources concerning the issues that need to be considered in the decision-making process in terms of practical and ethical decision making. These issues are also discussed in more detail in Chapter 13.

IRENE'S CASE

The motor neurones that stimulate the intercostal muscles, diaphragm and epiglottal closure may have become affected and cause poor lung expansion and the risk of silent aspiration. Her physical discomforts may indicate that she is suffering retention of carbon dioxide. She should be positioned and well supported by pillows at an angle of about 45 degrees. Minimise anxiety which will worsen hypercapnia by giving her information about what you are doing and why. Also teach her to do counted breathing, which may distract her from anxiety, calm her and allow her body to make better use of the available oxygen. If the blood reports show that the pCO_2 is above 5.5 then overnight pulse oximetry may give an oxygen saturation pattern that can be sent to the laboratory for analysis. It may be counterproductive to give oxygen since this may affect the respiratory drive adversely. If the breathing problem is very severe, very short term non-invasive positive pressure ventilation may help rebalance blood oxygen and carbon monoxide levels. The physiotherapist can assess her breathing function and demonstrate how to give an assisted cough. As breathing and swallowing are closely connected and involve some of the same cranial nerves, a speech and language therapist needs to thoroughly assess Irene's swallowing ability in order to prevent aspiration that might cause a chest infection and serious problems for her.

ANWAH'S CASE
Anwah is at risk of chest infection because of her reduced mobility and the presence of a tracheostomy tube. It may be helpful to use hyoscine patches to reduce loose secretions and send a sample of the sputum to microbiology. Side lying positional changes will aid drainage of secretions, with head and chest raised at angle above the abdomen. If measures are taken to thicken the secretions a little, ensure that the mucus does not become too thick and likely to form plugs. Physiotherapy treatment will help clear the secretions from deep in the lungs.

SUMMARY
❏ Neurological impairments can cause problems in regulating breathing and maintaining a clear airway. They arise from injury or insult to the cerebral cortex or brain stem as infarction or traumatic injury, or from inflammation or degeneration of the peripheral nerves affecting the efficacy of the muscles of respiration.
❏ Other homeostatic mechanisms affecting breathing rate and rhythm include carbon dioxide levels, blood temperature, irritation of airways, pain and strong emotion.
❏ Nursing assessment should include the breathing pattern, the efficiency of protective mechanisms, the strength and

power of the respiratory muscles in achieving adequate ventilation, and the risks of aspiration.

❏ Nursing interventions include correct positioning, preventing regurgitation, managing secretions, suctioning according to evidence-based guidelines.

❏ Care of a patient with a tracheostomy needs an evidence-based care plan that includes the frequency of cleaning and replacing the tracheostomy tube, the inner tube, the stoma dressing and the ties. The tenacity or looseness of the secretions needs to be carefully managed.

❏ Other members of the interdisciplinary team, such as physiotherapist and speech and language therapist, make skilled assessments and can suggest interventions that can be incorporated in the nursing care plan.

REFERENCES

Akgul, S. and Akyolcu, N. (2002) Effects of normal saline on endotracheal suctioning. *Journal of Clinical Nursing* **11** (6), 826–30.

Baker, L. (2001) Nursing ethical issues related to home based ventilation for people with motor neurone disease. *Australasian Journal of Neuroscience* **14** (1).

Blackwood, B. (1998) The practice and perception of intensive care staff using the closed system suctioning. *Journal of Advanced Nursing* **28** (5), 1020–9.

Blackwood, B. (1999) Normal saline instillation with endotracheal suctioning: primum non nocere (first do no harm). *Journal of Advanced Nursing* **29** (4), 928–34.

Buglass, E. (1999) Clinical tracheostomy care: tracheal suction and humidification. *British Journal of Nursing* **8** (8), 500–4.

Clarke, L. (1995) A critical event in tracheostomy care. *British Journal of Nursing* **4** (12), 676–81.

Day, T., Farnell, S. and Wilson-Barnett, J. (2002a) Suctioning: a review of current research recommendations. *Intensive and Critical Care Nursing* **18** (2), 79–89.

Day, T., Farnell, S., Hatnes, S., Wainwright, S. and Wilson-Barnett, J. (2002b) Tracheal suctioning: an exploration of nurses' knowledge and competence in acute and high dependency ward areas. *Journal of Advanced Nursing* **39** (1), 35–45.

Docherty, B. and Bench, S. (2002) Tracheostomy management for patients in general ward settings. *Professional Nurse* **18** (2), 100–4.

Ede, V. and McGowan, S. (2001) Tracheosotomy management revisited. *Nursing and Residential Care* **3** (3), 119–20, 122, 138–9.

Glass, C. and Grap, M. (1995) Ten tips for safe suctioning. *American Journal of Nursing* **5** (5), 51–3.

Gosselink, R., Kovacs, L., Ketelaer, P., Carton, H. and Decramer, M. (2000) Respiratory muscle weakness and respiratory muscle training in severely disabled multiple sclerosis patients. *Archives of Physical Medicine and Rehabilitation* **81** (6), 747–51.

Griggs, A. (1998) Tracheostomy: suctioning and humidification. *Nursing Standard* **13** (2), 49.

Hagler, D. and Traver, G. (1994) Endotracheal saline and suction catheters: sources of lower airway contamination. *American Journal of Critical Care* **3** (6), 444–7.

Harkin, H. and Russell, C. (2001) Tracheostomy patient care. *Nursing Times* **97** (25), 34–6.

Hayashi, H. and Oppenheimer, E. A. (2003) ALS patients on TPPV: totally locked in state, neurologic findings and ethical implications. *Neurology* **61** (1), 135–7.

Hilling, L. *et al.* (1992) Nasotracheal suctioning. *Respiratory Care* **37** (9), 898–901.

Jablonski, R. (1994) The experience of being mechanically ventilated. *Qualitative Health Research* **4** (2), 186–207.

Jamieson, E. M., McCall, J. M. and Whyte, L. A. (2002) *Clinical Nursing Practices*, 4th edn. Churchill Livingstone, Edinburgh.

Jevon, P. and Ewens, B. (2002) *Monitoring the Critically Ill Patient*. Blackwell Science, Oxford.

Kent, M. A. (1996) The ethical arguments concerning the artificial ventilation of patients with motor neurone disease. *Nursing Ethics* **3** (4), 318–27.

Kinloch, D. (1999) Instillation of normal saline during endotracheal suctioning: effects on mixed venous oxygen saturation. *American Journal of Critical Care* **8** (4), 231–40.

Laws-Chapman, C. (1998) How to guides: tracheostomy tube management. *Care of the Critically Ill* **14** (5), insert 4pp.

Luce, J., Pierson, D. and Tyler, M. (1993) *Intensive Respiratory Care*, 2nd edn. W.B. Saunders, Philadelphia.

Macmillan, C. (1995) Nasopharyngeal suction study reveals knowledge deficit. *Nursing Times* **91** (50), 28–30.

Mallet, J. and Dougherty, L. (2000) *The Royal Marsden NHS Trust Manual of Clinical Nursing Procedures*, 5th edn. Blackwell Science, Oxford.

MND Society (2004) *Saliva Control*, information sheet, available at http://www.mndassociation.org

Moore, T. (2003) Suctioning techniques for the removal of respiratory secretions. *Nursing Standard* **18** (9), 47–53.

Moss, A. H., Casey, P., Stocking, C. B., Roos, R. P., Brooks, B. R. and Seiger, M. (1993) Home ventilation for amyotropic lateral sclerosis patients. *Neurology* **43**, 438–43.

Neill, K. (2001) Normal saline instillation prior to endotracheal suction: a literature review. *Nursing in Critical Care* **6** (1), 34–9.

Oppenheimer, E. A. (1993) Decision-making in the respiratory care of amyotropic lateral sclerosis: should home mechanical ventilation be used? *Palliative Medicine* **7** (4), Supplement 2, 49–64.

Parker, L. (1999) Infection control 1: a practical guide to glove usage. *British Journal of Nursing* **8** (7), 716–20.

Place, B. and Fell, H. (1998) Clearing tracheobronchial secretions using suction. *Nursing Times* **94** (47), 54–6.

Peruzzi, W. T., Logemann, J. A., Currie, D. and Moen, S. G. (2001) Assessment of aspiration in patients with tracheostomies: comparison of the bedside coloured dye assessment with videofluoroscopic examination. *Respiratory Care* **46** (3), 243–7.

Serra, A. (2000) Tracheostomy care. *Nursing Standard* **14** (42), 45–52.

Spence, A. (1995) Home ventilation: how to plan for discharge. *Nursing Standard* **9** (42), 38–40.

Tamburri, L. M. (2000) Care of a patient with a tracheostomy. *Orthopaedic Nursing* **19** (2), 49–60.

Tantucci, C., Massucci, M., Piperno, R., Betti, L., Grassi, V. and Sorbibini, C. A. (1994) Control of breathing and respiratory muscle strength in patients with multiple sclerosis. *Chest* **105** (4), 1163–70.

Taylor-Piliae, R. (2002) Review: several techniques to optimise oxygenation during suctioning of patients. *Evidence-Based Nursing* **5** (2), 51.

Thompson, L. (2000) Suctioning adults with an artificial airway. *Systematic Review* **9**, The Joanna Briggs Institute for Nursing and Midwifery, Adelaide.

Weins, M. E., Reimer, M. A. and Guyn, H. L. (1999) Music therapy as a treatment method for improving respiratory muscle strength in patients with advanced multiple sclerosis: a pilot study. *Rehabilitation Nursing* **24** (2), 74–80.

Wainwright, S. P. and Gould, D. (1996) Endotracheal suctioning: an example of the problems of relevance and rigour in clinical research. *Journal of Clinical Nursing* **5**, 389–98.

Ward, V. *et al.* (1997) *Hospital Acquired Infection: Surveillance Policies and Practice. Preventing Hospital Acquired Infection: Clinical Guidelines.* Public Health Laboratory Service, London.

Wood, C. (1998) Endotracheal suctioning: a literature review. *Intensive and Critical Care Nursing* **14** (3), 124–36.

6 | Eating and Drinking

INTRODUCTION

Although water and nourishment are basic survival needs, the activity of eating and drinking assumes several other important functions in life. It has great social and cultural significance, and in most cultures is associated with friendship, hospitality, celebratory and ceremonial occasions. Psychological and emotional factors also play a part in influencing appetite and in shaping a person's eating and drinking habits, knowledge about diet and attitudes towards food and drink. People with neurological impairment may not be able to prepare their own meals, they may have difficulty swallowing which affects the type of food they can eat and which may cause them social embarrassment because of coughing, spluttering or drooling. They may experience fatigue and they may not feel much like eating if they are low in mood. These problems can occur in several neurological conditions, such as stroke, bleeding from a cerebral vessel, multiple sclerosis, Parkinson's disease, dementia, myasthenia gravis and motor neurone disease. Malnutrition is common in neurological conditions, and in stroke patients often worsens during the first week or two following admission and can affect the overall outcome (RCP 2002; MAG 2003). This chapter focuses on how to meet the needs of patients at risk of malnutrition, patients with swallowing problems, patients who are fed enterally and the implications that might have for the administration of medicines. These aspects have been selected because they are frequently encountered in neurological patients and involve core skills in meeting patients' nutritional needs orally or through a tube.

LEARNING OUTCOMES

❏ Outline the stages of swallowing and the risk factors, signs and symptoms of dysphagia.

❏ Awareness of protocols and guidelines for swallowing screen and for implementing nutritional support for patients with neurological damage.

❏ Describe principles of effective assistance, including psychological and emotional effects of altered style and patterns of eating, the use of adapted utensils, feeding technique and food consistency estimation.

❏ Describe safe practices in enteral feeding and medication through nasogastric or percutaneous routes.

❏ Appreciate ethical issues in initiating and withdrawing nutritional support.

FACTORS AFFECTING NUTRITION

The healthy human body is reasonably well able to support periods of starvation (although not dehydration) with little clinical effect evident, with a weight loss of approximately 10% over a period of ten days (Leary *et al.* 2000). However, people who are acutely or critically ill have a stress response that speeds up the metabolic rate, which plunders all body tissue, including protein mass, and leads to more rapid deterioration and malnutrition. In the acute stage of an illness this can quickly manifest as:

• delayed wound healing;
• increased vulnerability to pressure sores;
• reduced resistance to infection;
• increased susceptibility to complications;
• increased mortality.

In people who have a long-term neurological problem, with prolonged inadequate intake over several months, the effects are more insidious and less visible because slower. In this adaptive phase to malnutrition, the body uses body fat and the resulting ketosis helps to conserve muscle protein and provides the brain with its main source of energy. In this type of starvation, the results may only be noticed as abnormal blood values.

There will be:

- increased breakdown of body fat;
- slow weight loss;
- slow loss of muscle mass;
- metabolic acidosis that is usually compensated for by respiratory alkalosis;
- lowered metabolic rate and body temperature;
- increased fluid retention and peripheral oedema (Hickey 1997).

The depletion of the body's resources exacerbates the fatigue that neurological patients often suffer, and worsens their condition, leading into a vicious circle.

COMMON NEUROLOGICAL IMPAIRMENTS THAT MAY LEAD TO MALNUTRITION

- Altered levels of consciousness.
- Impaired cognition, such as attention span, memory problems, orientation and judgement problems affecting contextual grasp of the situation as well as the reflex swallowing process.
- Impaired motor ability, with reduced rate, strength and range of motion of the lips, tongue, jaw movement, poor peristalsis through pharynx, and impairment of closure of epiglottis and oesophageal reflux.
- Impaired sensation in the mouth and cheeks leading to pocketing of food, and impaired sensation in the pharynx leading to delayed swallow.
- Impaired vision or perception such as hemianopia.
- Impaired motor ability of arms.

All the characters in the case studies (see section on How to Use this Book) have impairments that could lead to malnutrition. Harry's restlessness and wandering will use up energy. Mark, even though his appetite is insatiable, may not have a balanced nutritional intake. Irene is showing signs of hypoxaemia related to her motor neurone disease and she may have impaired swallowing function. Miriam needs to be eating a nutritional diet if she is to have her PEG removed and she may need close monitoring to see if food is pocketing in her mouth.

Louise needs to eat a healthy low-fat, high-fibre diet with plenty of fruit and vegetables to combat fatigue and reduce chance of constipation developing. If her upper limbs are affected, she will not have precision of fine movement. Anwah is clearly dependent on others to help her meet her nutritional needs, but she also needs adequate water intake in addition to her feeds. Gary has postural problems that could interfere with eating, and his right arm, which may be his utensil-holding arm, is contracted. Joyce has to come to terms with eating a soft diet and thickened fluids, and Ella has both swallowing problems and a dense weakness of her right side, which will affect utensil control. She may even have visual problems locating the food on her plate. She is a well-covered woman and clearly must have eaten with gusto before her stroke. Fred may have difficulty eating if the muscles of his throat and neck are affected and because of the limitation of his movement.

Table 6.1 sets out the common risk factors that can cause swallowing or nutritional deficits.

MECHANISM OF SWALLOWING

Successful swallowing is dependent on the proper functioning of six cranial nerves. These co-ordinate sensory information about the presence of material at the lips, in the mouth and in the pharynx. They also co-ordinate the muscles needed to move the material safely through the mouth, pharynx and oesophagus. In addition, they protect the body from the material entering the airways and lungs through coughing, or protect the stomach from noxious material through gagging. Co-ordinated swallowing activity is, however, much more than coughing or gagging. The stages of swallowing are shown in Figure 6.1.

The assessment of swallowing should not be confused with eliciting the following simple reflexes, although, when impaired, these reflexes can cause choking or silent aspiration.

- *Cough reflex* is a protective reflex that prevents food from entering the airways. In neurological disease, it can be diminished or ineffective.
- *Gag reflex* protects the digestive system by preparing the body to eject noxious material from entering the digestive tract.

Table 6.1 Common risk factors which can cause swallowing or nutritional deficits.

	Altered sensation	Altered motor ability	Altered cognition/perception
Stroke	Diminshed sensation to trigger swallow reflex Hemianopia	Weakness of muscles of mastication Postural changes Hemiparesis Altered sitting balance	Altered level of consciousness Oral apraxia
Traumatic brain injury	Diminished sensation to trigger swallow reflex	Weakness of muscles of mastication. Increased activity states/motor restlessness	Distractability Memory impairment Short attention span Altered level of consciousness Agitation
Parkinson's disease		Diminished motor swallow Postural/head position disturbance Inability to control secretions	Levodopa less effective if high protein diet taken
Multiple sclerosis		Spasticity of trunk and limb	Visual disturbance Depth perception
Epilepsy		Choking if seizure activity occurs while eating	Some anticonvulsants may interfere with B complex absorption Seizure activity may interfere with memory
Dementia	May lose sense of taste, ability to recognise taste	Extra calorie needs if agitated and wandering	May forget to eat Confabulate eating behaviour May suspect others of trying to poison
Motor neurone disease		Muscles of mastication become weak Swallowing co-ordination may fail	

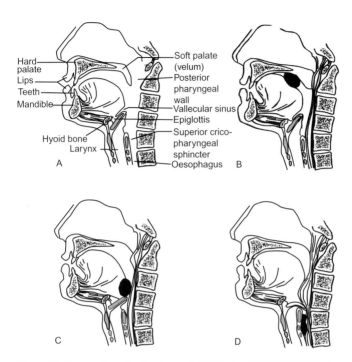

Hard palate
Lips
Teeth
Mandible
Hyoid bone
Larynx
Soft palate (velum)
Posterior pharyngeal wall
Vallecular sinus
Epiglottis
Superior crico-pharyngeal sphincter
Oesophagus
A
B
C
D

Figure 6.1 Stages of swallowing. B = oral phase; C = pharyngeal phase; D = oesophageal phase. Reproduced with permission (Hickey 1997).

Swallowing is a complicated act that usually begins voluntarily, but is always completed by reflex. The common practice of touching the fauces to elicit a gag reflex is *not* indicative of a swallowing reflex.

Nurses can make a significant contribution to a patient's nutritional plan of care by carrying out an early swallowing screen assessment (see Figure 6.2) to identify patients at risk of inadequate intake or silent aspiration. During a multicentre study in six UK hospitals in which nurses were trained to use a swallowing screen assessment, the proportion of patients with unsafe swallowing in whom no precautions were taken against aspiration was reduced by two-thirds (Ellul *et al.* 1997). Any patient with an abnormal swallow should be treated according

WITH PATIENT ALERT AND SAT UPRIGHT:

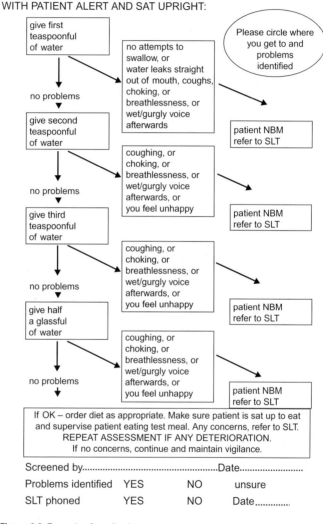

give first teaspoonful of water

Please circle where you get to and problems identified

no attempts to swallow, or water leaks straight out of mouth, coughs, choking, or breathlessness, or wet/gurgly voice afterwards

no problems

patient NBM refer to SLT

give second teaspoonful of water

coughing, or choking, or breathlessness, or wet/gurgly voice afterwards, or you feel unhappy

no problems

patient NBM refer to SLT

give third teaspoonful of water

coughing, or choking, or breathlessness, or wet/gurgly voice afterwards, or you feel unhappy

no problems

patient NBM refer to SLT

give half a glassful of water

coughing, or choking, or breathlessness, or wet/gurgly voice afterwards, or you feel unhappy

no problems

patient NBM refer to SLT

coughing, or choking, or breathlessness, or wet/gurgly voice afterwards, or you feel unhappy

patient NBM refer to SLT

If OK – order diet as appropriate. Make sure patient is sat up to eat and supervise patient eating test meal. Any concerns, refer to SLT. REPEAT ASSESSMENT IF ANY DETERIORATION. If no concerns, continue and maintain vigilance.

Screened by...Date.......................

Problems identified   YES   NO   unsure

SLT phoned   YES   NO   Date..............

Figure 6.2 Example of swallowing screen.

> **Box 6.1 National guidelines for good practice in the assessment and management of dysphagia and nutrition (RCP 1999)**
>
> - All patients should have their swallow assessed as soon as possible by appropriately trained personnel using a simple validated bedside testing protocol.
> - Any patient with abnormal swallow should be seen by a speech and language therapist who should assess further and advise the patient and staff on safe swallow and consistency of diet and fluids.
> - Every patient should have his or her nutritional status screened by appropriately trained personnel using a valid nutritional screening method within 48 hours of admission.
> - Nutritional support should be considered in any malnourished patient.
> - Percutaneous endoscopic gastrostomy (PEG) tubes (or nasogastric tubes) where patients are unable to maintain adequate nutrition orally.
> - Every patient with nutritional problems, including dysphagia, which requires food of modified consistency should be referred to a dietician.
> - Patients' needs should be assessed for the most suitable posture and equipment to facilitate feeding.

---

to the recommendations for good practice as identified by the Royal College of Physicians (RCP 1999) – see Box 6.1.

RISK FACTORS, SIGNS AND SYMPTOMS OF DYSPHAGIA

Oral phase (see Figure 6.1B)
- Poor lip closure
- Drooling
- Pocketing of food
- Oral weakness with reduced sensitivity
- Poor tongue control
- Inability to start and transport food to the back of the mouth

- Uncoordinated or excessive chewing
- Multiple swallows for each mouthful

Pharyngeal phase (see Figure 6.1C)
- Inadequate sealing between pharynx and larynx, with coughing and spluttering
- Frequent clearing of throat
- Delayed swallowing reflex
- Absence of cough reflex
- Changes in the voice quality, with wet, gurgling sound in voice

Oesophageal phase (see Figure 6.1D)
- Burping
- Substernal distress
- Coughing or wheezing

ELLA'S CASE
A dysphagia trained nurse and a speech and language therapist should assess the extent of Ella's swallowing problems. This can only take place when Ella is alert and is supported to sit in an upright position. If Ella is able to take a modified diet, the nurse should be vigilant and monitor closely for any change in Ella's chest, breathing or temperature. If any abnormalities are observed, oral intake should be withheld. The nurse should also be observant for any further changes in this activity, for example increased drooling and gurgly, wet sounding speech. If food pockets on the right side of her mouth the nurse should clear this using a sweep with gloved finger, or inform Ella how to clear this herself. Correct mouth care is also of high importance as post-stroke patients often develop oral thrush due to decreased fluid intake. The nurse should also maintain an accurate fluid balance chart to ensure Ella does not become dehydrated.

ASSESSMENT AND CARE PLANNING
In assessment, nurses need to know about the person's normal eating habits and attitudes towards food and to take into account their psychological and emotional responses to the changes that may have taken place in their eating and drinking

patterns and styles since the onset of neurological problems. Miriam's apparent reluctance to eat might be because of low mood – a frequent sign of depression – or it could be related to perceptual or cognitive impairments of her brain injury, or it could be that she has always been fussy about what she eats. Louise may have financial concerns, and she economises on food, or she may have body image disturbances because of her concerns about her sexual attractiveness. Within the context of a holistic assessment, some units have developed nutritional assessment sheets. An example is shown in Figure 6.3. Nutritional assessment needs to be a team endeavour, although nurses have the responsibility of early detection of groups at risk. The nutritional assessment should include physical observations of the patient's appearance and weight, identification of risk factors as well as a swallowing screen, and evaluation of blood results from the laboratory (Hickey 1997). Once an agreed nutritional plan has been made with the patient, physician, speech and language therapist, dietician and pharmacist, the role of the nurse is to:

- provide, as far as possible, an environment in which the person feels comfortable eating, food that is to their liking in portions suitable for their appetite and of an appropriate texture and consistency;
- monitor indicators of nutritional state by weighing the patient and noting trends, observing skin turgor and body muscle tone and monitoring and recording fluid balance and nutritional intake;
- select, monitor and maintain any modified eating utensils or other feeding equipment used;
- monitor the tolerance of enteral feeding following local protocols on aspirating a feeding tube;
- monitor the patient's activity level and fatigue.

SERVING FOOD AND USING MODIFIED UTENSILS AND EATING EQUIPMENT

At first, people may be deeply embarrassed by their need for special utensils or the need to have food cut or puréed. With tact and time this can resolve. Tact includes cutting up food in

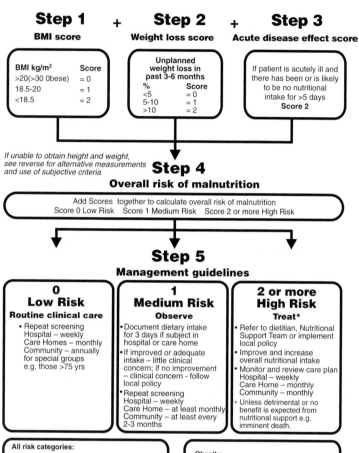

Step 1 + Step 2 + Step 3

BMI score   **Weight loss score**   **Acute disease effect score**

BMI kg/m²	Score
>20(>30 0bese)	= 0
18.5-20	= 1
<18.5	= 2

Unplanned weight loss in past 3-6 months

%	Score
<5	= 0
5-10	= 1
>10	= 2

If patient is acutely ill and there has been or is likely to be no nutritional intake for >5 days
Score 2

If unable to obtain height and weight, see reverse for alternative measurements and use of subjective criteria

Step 4
Overall risk of malnutrition

Add Scores together to calculate overall risk of malnutrition
Score 0 Low Risk   Score 1 Medium Risk   Score 2 or more High Risk

Step 5
Management guidelines

0 Low Risk
Routine clinical care

- Repeat screening
  Hospital – weekly
  Care Homes – monthly
  Community – annually
  for special groups
  e.g. those >75 yrs

1 Medium Risk
Observe

- Document dietary intake for 3 days if subject in hospital or care home
- If improved or adequate intake – little clinical concern; if no improvement – clinical concern - follow local policy
- Repeat screening
  Hospital – weekly
  Care Home – at least monthly
  Community – at least every 2-3 months

2 or more High Risk
Treat*

- Refer to dietitian, Nutritional Support Team or implement local policy
- Improve and increase overall nutritional intake
- Monitor and review care plan
  Hospital – weekly
  Care Home – monthly
  Community – monthly
- Unless detrimental or no benefit is expected from nutritional support e.g. imminent death.

All risk categories:
- Treat underlying condition and provide help and advice on food choices, eating and drinking when necessary.
- Record malnutrition risk category.
- Record need for special diets and follow local policy.

Obesity:
- Record presence of obesity. For those with underlying conditions, these are generally controlled before the treatment of obesity.

Re-assess subjects identified at risk as they move through care settings
See The 'MUST' Explanatory Booklet for further details and The 'MUST' Report for supporting evidence.

Figure 6.3 Reproduced with permission of the Malnutrition Advisory Group (MAG), which is a standing committee of BAPEN (www.bapen.org).

the kitchen before serving it to the patient. This overcomes the potentially humiliating experience for the person of publicly having their food cut up. If the food is puréed, it should preferably be served in moulds that resemble the shape of the food, or at least served in separate servings to preserve colour appeal.

Patients should also be encouraged to use a serviette or napkin in whatever way they feel is most useful and dignified for them. Some may choose to protect their clothes from the neck down; others may prefer to use it more discreetly. Nurses can also discuss with patients a range of different utensils they could try such as enlarged or built-up handles on utensils make grasping easier for patients with fine motor deficits. The handle can be lengthened or bent for people with reduced range of motion, and a rocker knife or combined spoon and fork can be provided to people with only one functioning hand. Small-diameter glasses made of unbreakable material may be appreciated by people with grasp deficits, and a friction or non-skid surface and plate guard can be useful for people who have difficulty controlling their movements. Drinking cups with handles large enough to insert the fingers may be useful, as might a long straw for people with limited range of movement. Examples of special utensils are given in Box 6.2.

MIRIAM'S CASE

Nurses need to look at Miriam from both a physical and a psychological perspective. She has not eaten or taken oral fluids for a long time. Are there any problems with oral hygiene, oral infection or ill-fitting dentures? Dental hygiene is very important and can be carried out using a Yankauer suction tube and ordinary toothbrush and toothpaste if the teeth are her own, or using proprietary denture cleaner in clean water if not. Is she carrying out activities to give her an appetite? If her rehabilitation is progressing well she should be getting hungry. If she appears not to have an appetite is this because of her emotional or psychological state of mind? Is she low in mood as a normal part of coming to terms with what has happened to her and with a changed body image, leading to a dependency she associates with babies and children? Does she fear that she may choke, or that she may eat clumsily, make a mess and

---

Box 6.2 Examples of adapted utensils

- Large-handled utensils: to help grasp for people with weakened grasp or spasticity.
- Long-handled utensils: to help people with limited shoulder and elbow movements.
- Plate guards: circular ring that attaches to a plate, prevents spills and assists loading of food on to utensil.
- Bent handles for people with limited range of motion. This may be in conjunction with extended and enlarged handles.
- Rocker knife or spoon and fork combined may be used by people with only one functioning hand.
- Swivel spoons.
- Utensil cuff surrounds the hand and has a slot for utensils for people with diminshed hand strength.
- Small-diameter glasses for people with limited grasp.
- Low-skid or friction mat under plate to prevent slip for people using one hand or who have uncontrolled movements.
- Cups with handles large enough to insert fingers to facilitate grasp.

---

embarrass herself? Is she having seizure activity that is affecting her levels of awareness and concentration? In addition, what kind of eater is she normally? Does she take frequent snacks and is she a grazer? Does she have strong preferences or a particularly sweet tooth ?

Nurses can assist Miriam to eat independently using a number of different approaches. Finger foods may offer her independence in feeding, as can soup or thickened fluids in a mug rather than food on a plate. If the food needs to be puréed, use moulds to ensure that the shape and colour are preserved. As the diet progresses towards different food textures, meat can be cut up in the kitchen before giving it to her. This can overcome the feeling of humiliation some people have as nurses stand over them and cut up their food. As the food is served, tell her what is on the plate and ask if it is to her liking. Offer a napkin and check that she is sitting in a comfortable position suitable for eating. Place adapted eating utensils or equipment discreetly. If she seems to want to be fed and you are not sure if she has a visual impairment, sit down next to her and give her verbal information about what type of food is on the plate and brush her lips gently with the utensil to prompt her to open her mouth and take a mouthful. Sometimes, if the appetite is small, teaspoons or dessert forks may provide suitably small mouthfuls.

Distractibility may be interfering with Miriam's concentration, which can often happen after brain injury. One way of prioritising good nutrition for all patients is to develop protected meal times. This means that at meal times all staff are dedicated to the activity, which means no interruptions such as telephone calls, meetings or non-essential clinical work.

FEEDING TECHNIQUES

Some patients will need physical assistance to eat. Good principles (Davies 1999; Joanna Briggs Institute 2000) of feeding include:

- Ensure patient is in upright position in 90 degree angle and that the person who is feeding should be at or below the patients eye level when feeding.
- Use sensible utensils as near normal as possible.
- Warn the patient verbally that the food is coming or brush the lips to stimulate mouth opening, and avoid touching the teeth or placing the food too far back in the mouth.
- Encourage small bites and frequent chewing.
- If fatigue is a problem, give six small meals a day rather than three large ones. This may involve the help of volunteers or family members if staffing is a problem.
- Place food in the unaffected side of the mouth if there is paralysis on one side.
- Check patient's mouth or ask patient to check for pocketing after each swallow by sweeping the mouth with a finger if safe to do so.
- Check if a speech and language therapist has recommended special techniques. These may include:

- techniques using head position to facilitate swallowing (see Box 6.3);
- techniques aimed at compensating for swallowing impairments (see Box 6.4);
- modified consistencies of fluids or food (see Table 6.2);
- tongue exercises;
- suctioning of oral secretions (see Chapter 5);
- thermal stimulation, 'icing' and use of tart tastes to stimulate saliva;
- use of special utensils (see Box 6.2), palatal lift prosthesis, special head and chin position, tilt and turn at pharyngeal stage, use of chin support during feeding. Examples of these positional strategies can be seen in Box 6.3.

Food consistencies can often be ambiguous and different members of staff may interpret food consistencies and fluid thickening descriptors differently. In order to overcome this it is advisable that there is certainly locally agreed terminology. The Royal College of Speech and Language Therapists and the British Dietetic Association have collaborated to produce guidance on reaching a consensus. These can be seen in Table 6.2.

All of these measures should ensure that patients at risk of aspiration and malnutrition from neurologically related problems are identified early, supported appropriately and maintain the best nutritional level possible by the most effective mode. Nutritional supplements may also be given where adequate nutritional intake is a problem.

ENTERAL NUTRITION

Enteral nutrition refers to nutrition support delivered through a tube to the stomach, duodenum or jejunum. It has become a widely used health care technology in critical and acute care, general hospital wards, nursing homes and in the community. Enteral tube feeding has increased in the community over the past few years, with an estimate that at any one point in time, over 10 000 patients receive enteral tube feeding in the community, which is over twice the number in hospital (Elia 1998).

Box 6.3 Compensatory treatment techniques (Davies 1999, reproduced with permission)

Change posture

Postural changes are compensatory measures, which facilitate the patients swallowing ability and are primarily determined by the speech and language therapist during videofluoroscopy examination. Typically the patient tries different head positions during the videofluoroscopy to determine which position gives the safest swallow.

Tilt chin down (chin tuck)

Frequently patients presenting with delayed triggering of the pharyngeal swallow can benefit from tilting the chin down into what is called the chin tuck position. This position usually widens the vallecular space, thus allowing the material to travel at a slower rate through the pharynx.

This technique can also be used for patients who experience reduced laryngeal closure, because the widened vallecuulae may divert material away from the laryngeal vestibule thus decreasing the risk of aspiration. Tilting the head down can be helpful with patients who have reduced base retraction. This position may allow for closer approximation of the tongue base to the pharyngeal wall during the pharyngeal phase of swallowing, thus creating increased pharyngeal pressure to propel the bolus through the pharynx.

Note that tilting the chin down may not be helpful in patients with reduced epiglottic function. These patients tend to retain vallecular residue since the epiglottis may fail to invert properly to allow the material to flow through pharynx. They are typically at risk of aspiration due to reduced or absent protection of the airway.

Turning the head to left/right

This can be useful to individuals who have unilateral pharyngeal paresis or paralysis. By turning the head towards the affected side, the bolus is propelled down the stronger side of the pharynx while bypassing the weaker vallecular and pyriform sinus. This reduces the amount of residue in the pharynx and decreases the risk for aspiration.

Continued

Turning the head to left/right with chin tuck
Patients with unilateral pharyngeal paresis or paralysis and a delayed triggering of the pharyngeal swallow may benefit from this compensatory position. Rotating the head to the affected side and tilting the chin down simultaneously will allow the material to flow through the stronger side of the pharynx, yet at a slower rate, which allows triggering of the pharyngeal swallow.

Tilt head to left and right
Patients with unilateral pharyngeal and/or lingual paralysis may benefit from tilting the head towards the stronger side of the pharynx. This allows the bolus to travel through the less affected side of the oral cavity and pharynx via gravitational pull. Note that the patient should have the head tilted towards the less affected side as food is placed in the mouth, otherwise the food may fall to the weaker side during the swallow, thus reducing the effectiveness of the compensatory strategy.

Change volume of food
Generally the bolus is reduced to increase the ability to swallow safely and easily. However, because of reduced sensation it can sometimes be necessary, particularly in older patients, to have a large bolus to trigger the swallow reflex.

Change food consistency
The use of thickened fluids can be helpful for people who have a delayed swallow. Thickened fluids tend to travel at a slower rate through the oral cavity and pharynx, allowing more time for the triggering of the pharyngeal swallow. Puréed diet is recommended for patients who can tolerate 'pudding consistency' or blended food. This is recommended for patients exhibiting difficulty with oral preparatory or oral stage of swallowing or a delayed swallow. Because of its uniform consistency it can help reduce the problem of material falling into the pharynx at different intervals, particularly when the patient is chewing.

Box 6.4 Basic principles of managing dysphagia (Bryce Evans *et al.* 1998)

Oral stage

Patients may not be able to chew or keep saliva in the mouth, and food and liquid may be aspirated before the swallow.

• Use multiple swallows, head positioning and strengthening muscles in the oral as well as the pharyngeal areas in patients with too much saliva.
• Use synthetic saliva with patients who have too little.
• Teach posterior tongue exercises and proper bolus placements to patients who have difficulty timing bolus transport and the tongue position and movement during swallow.
• Exercise the tongue and lips to increase their movement range and strength during mastication.

Pharyngeal stage

• Use ice or highly flavoured products for patients with reduced pharyngeal sensation.
• Use of trigger reflex techniques such as thermal stimulation. A refrigerated laryngeal mirror is touched to the base of the anterior faucial arch several times, which in time may stimulate the swallow reflex.
• Teach supraglottic swallow. The patients takes a breath, holds it, swallows and coughs one or more times immediately after swallowing. This dislodges any material remaining in the hypopharynx and prevents the patient from ingesting the material immediately after swallowing.
• Tilt the head forward and down. This will widen the valleculae and bring the epiglottis forward, protecting the airway.
• Adjust the bolus size and provide thermal stimulation to help correct such timing problems as delayed swallow initiation.
• Reposition and alter posture, such as head tilts and chin tucks (see Box 6.2).
• Medical management such as botulinum toxin.

Table 6.2 Texture Modification – fluid (RCSLT/BDA 2003).

Texture	Description of fluid texture	Example
Thin fluid	Still water	Water, tea, coffee without milk, diluted squash, spirits, wine
Naturally thick fluid	Product leaves a coating on an empty glass	Full cream milk, cream liqueurs, Complan, Build Up (made to instructions) Nutriment, commercial sip feeds
Thickened fluid	Fluid to which a commercial thickener has been added to thicken consistency	
Stage 1	• Can be drunk through a straw • Can be drunk from a cup if advised or preferred • Leaves a thin coat on the back of the spoon	
Stage 2	• Cannot be drunk through a straw • Can be drunk from a cup • Leaves a thick coat on the back of the spoon	
Stage 3	• Cannot be drunk through a straw • Cannot be drunk from a cup • Needs to be taken with a spoon	

Dysphagia, which may be related to cerebrovascular accident, multiple sclerosis, motor neurone disease or brain injury (Parker *et al.* 1996), is probably the most common reason for initiating enteral feeding. Early establishment of an enteral feeding regime is important in moving acutely ill patients from the catabolic state, and in protecting the linings of the digestive tract from the risk of stress ulcers. Early feeding also helps to prevent the movement of harmful bacteria from the gastrointestinal tract to the bloodstream through a mucosal barrier that is compromised by low blood flow and relative ischaemia (Anderton 1995; Kennedy 1997; Wood *et al.* 1997; Leary *et al.* 2000; Dorman 2003). In addition, Metheny (1996) established associations between feeding and improved gut function, enhanced immune function, reduced infection rates and better survival rates in the critically ill.

Nasogastric/nasojejunal/nasoduodenal feeding is commonly used for short-term needs and can be used with unconscious patients in the initial stages of trauma or brain injury where good nutrition enhances recovery and can prevent the development of stress ulcers. Fine bore tubes are more comfortable for patients and are less likely to cause complications such as irritation of gastrointestinal tract. In addition, the use of drugs such as cisapride or metaclopromide can aid the tolerance and absorption of enteral feeds (Adam 1994, Ball 1994, Zainal 1994). However, neurological patients with longer-term swallowing problems will opt for gastrostomy feeding.

Gastrostomy or jejunostomy feeding (PEG or PEJ) is given through a tube that is placed through a small incision in the abdominal wall with the help of an endoscope, usually under local anaesthetic. PEG tubes vary in size from 9 FG to 28 FG and last up to two years. They come in a range of different types, with the choice usually based on efficacy, cost/benefit considerations and estimated period of feeding.

Current recommendations (Mallett and Dougherty 2000) suggest that pump-assisted delivery is the most effective administration, commencing with a full-strength feed at a low rate of 25–30 ml per hour. The choice between intermittent or continuous infusion needs to be discussed with the patient, nurses and carers, bearing in mind the advantages and disadvantages shown in Table 6.3. Some evidence suggests that overnight feeding can improve nutrition by allowing increased supplementary intake during the day (Bastow *et al.* 1985) and facilitating weaning.

Trouble shooting feeding problems

Several sources (Kennedy 1997, Collier 2004, Elia *et al.* 1994) indicate that speech and language therapists, dieticians and

Table 6.3 Methods of administering enteral feeds (Mallett and Dougherty 2000, with permission from Blackwell Publishing).

Feeding regime	Advantages	Disadvantages
Continuous feeding via a pump	Easily controlled rate Reduction of gastrointestinal complications	Patient connected to tube for the majority of the day May limit patient's mobility
Intermittent feeding via gravity or pump	Periods of time free of feeding Flexible feeding routine May be easier than managing a pump for some patients	May have an increased risk of gastrointestinal symptoms, e.g. early satiety Difficult if outside carers are involved with the feed
Bolus feeding	May reduce time connected to the feed Very easy Minimum equipment needed	May have increased risk of gastrointestinal symptoms Can be time consuming

pharmacists should be included in the multidisciplinary team to help establish effective regimes and to troubleshoot problems. Conscientious monitoring of patients and clinical reasoning can detect changes that might indicate a problem early, such as in Table 6.4; and prompt intervention prevents the problem from developing fully. In addition to the laboratory results, electrolyte disturbances can be picked up by alterations in the urine output, in the patient's behaviour and muscle strength, and in the stool output (Metheny 1996).

Mouth care

In addition to those who have no oral intake, some patients may have decreased mastication and saliva or excess saliva. The shape of the mouth may have changed; dentures may rub in places or may no longer fit properly. There may be sensory disturbance and food or tablets may lodge in the cheek or against the gums and cause local irritation. Some patients may also have lost some cognitive ability and have memory and concentration loss, and need supervision or prompting with oral

Table 6.4 Potential problems with administration of feed (Crest 2004, with permission).

Problem	Cause	Intervention
Nausea and vomiting	Feeding position of the patient	Ensure head and shoulders are raised to an angle of approximately 30 degrees during feeding and for at least one hour after feeding stops. Consider daytime feeding
	Intestinal obstruction	Observe the patient for signs of abdominal distention. Refer patient to doctor urgently for assessment
	Hyperosmolar feed – rapid infusion rate	Ask dietician to review feed and feeding regime
	Delayed gastric emptying	Observe the patient for signs of abdominal discomfort or distention. Refer to the doctor for monitoring of same and consideration of gut motility drugs. If problem persists it may be necessary to consider feeding beyond the stomach into the jejunum, therefore refer the patient back to the endoscopist or gastroenterologist
	Side effect of medication	Review medication with doctor and or pharmacist and consider alternative treatment
Aspiration	Swallowing difficulties	Stop all oral intake. Refer patient to speech and language therapist for advice regarding oral intake. Refer patient to dentist for assessment, considerable care now required with toothbrushing – dentist will advise

Table 6.4 *Continued*

Problem	Cause	Intervention
	Position of the feeding tube/position of the patient	Check that the tip of the feeding tube is in the correct place . Ensure head and shoulders are raised to an angle of approximately 30 degrees during feeding and for at least one hour after feeding stops. Consider daytime feeding
	Delayed gastric emptying	Observe the patient for signs of abdominal discomfort or distention. Discuss with dietician and consider reduction of volume of feed/fluid administration, i.e. changing the type of feed. Refer to the doctor for monitoring of same and consideration of gut motility drugs. If problem persists it may be necessary to consider feeding beyond the stomach into the jejunum, therefore refer the patient back to the endoscopist or gastroenterologist
Diarrhoea	Pre-existing bowel disorder	Review medical history and consider previous bowel pattern
	Side effect of medication	Discuss with doctor or pharmacist and consider alternative medication and or the use of antidiarrhoeals
	Infection	Send specimen of faeces to bacteriology for culture and sensitivity. Ensure the appropriate infection control measures are in place and review handling of the feed, feeding system and accessory feeding equipment
	Feed	Discuss type of feed and rate of administration with dietician
Constipation	Low residue feed	Discuss change to fibre-enhanced feed residue with dietician
	Inadequate fluid intake	Check patient is receiving all feed and fluid prescribed. Ensure accurate record kept on fluid balance chart if appropriate. Consider patient biochemistry and consider increasing patient fluid requirements, especially if patient has pyrexia or during hot weather
	Side effect of medication	Discuss with doctor or pharmacist and consider the use of laxatives

hygiene. Mouth care should be assessed and planned as part of nutritional care to prevent caries, mouth infection and soreness, dry and cracked lips and halitosis.

Miriam, for example, seems to be reluctant to eat and there could be a host of reasons, ranging from mood to perceptual and cognitive problems, but it may also be something fairly simple such as a sore mouth or ill-fitting dentures. A speech and language therapist may be able to offer suggestions about oral hygiene and a referral to a dentist should give a thorough assessment of any problems in the mouth.

MANAGING DRUG THERAPY IN ENTERAL NUTRITION

Thompson *et al.* (2000) note that several surveys highlight deficiencies in knowledge among nursing staff who routinely give drugs via a nasogastric tube, despite the fact that the nursing profession as a whole has demonstrated significant interest in the field in publications. In a study of all drug-related absorption problems, the most frequent problems concerned drug interactions with enteral or parenteral nutrition and inappropriate administration techniques (Cerulli and Malone 1999). The pharmacist can advise on how to prevent such problems (see Box 6.5), and nurses should consult them when enteral feeding is initiated. Considerations include the formulation to be used, whether any interaction with the feed may occur, the type of tube and placement site and the site of drug absorption (Thompson *et al.* 2000). In many cases this may lead to suggestions of alternatives to the enteral route, examples of which are shown in Box 6.6. In addition certain drugs common in neurological nursing need adjustments to dosage or frequency (see Table 6.5).

Drug formulations used in enteral feeding

* *Liquids, elixirs, suspensions or syrups.* It is wise to check with a pharmacist on the suitability of the formulation for enteral feeds (Jamieson *et al.* 2002). Some liquids are too viscous (Havard and Tiziani 1994); syrups can be too acidic or the sorbitol content or osmolality may cause diarrhoea, bloating or stomach cramps.

- *Soluble or dispersible tablets.* These may be used if a liquid preparation is unsuitable or unavailable.
- *Crushed tablets.* A list of tablets which should not be crushed may be available. In addition, the crushing of delayed-release tablets may result in dangerous peaks of drug activity. Enteric-coated tablets should not be crushed either, since the purpose of the coating is to protect the stomach and the particles may block the feeding tube (Thompson *et al.* 2000)
- *Capsule contents.* If all else fails, the possibility of opening capsules and flushing their contents down the tube can be explored, but this does carry a high risk of blocking the tube.

Box 6.5 Role of the pharmacist in managing patients on artificial nutrition

- Advising on suitable routes of drug administration, formulation or alternative preparations.
- Advising on medication timing and alerting nursing staff to drugs which may have to be given outside the routine drug rounds.
- Monitoring for loss of efficacy or toxicity due to drug interactions with feeds and reduced absorption owing to feeding tube site etc.
- Educating nursing staff about administration techniques and contributing to in-service training.
- Liaising with the multidisciplinary team to identify patients requiring pharmacist input, producing local guidelines, auditing of administration techniques.
- Discharge planning liaison between hospital and community pharmacies over fomulation, etc.
- Educating patient or carer about appropriate administration techniques.
- Providing back-up information.

Box 6.6 Suggested alternatives to enteral route for selected drugs (based on Thompson *et al.* 2000)

- *Intravenous* – usually the most expensive; requires trained staff and potentially prone to complications.
- *Intramuscular* – e.g. fosphenytoin.
- *Subcutaneous injection or infusion* – opioids, anti-emetics, and anxyiolitic combinations.
- *Transdermal* – glyceryl trinitrate patches, morphine patches.
- *Sublingual* – sublingual lorezepam, nifedepine.
- *Buccal* – buccal glyceral trinitrate, anti-emetics.
- *Rectal* – diclofenac, aspirin, diazepam, carbemezepine, laxative suppositories.

Table 6.5 Drugs requiring dosage or frequency adjustments when administered via enteral feeding tubes (adapted from Thompson *et al.* 2000).

Drug	Adjustment
Carbamezepine	Use suppositories available as 125 mg, 250 mg (125 mg rectally is approximately equivalent to 100 mg carbamezepine orally)
Levodopa (Madopar)	When changing to dispersible tablets total daily dose may need to be given more frequently. For controlled release formulations, 400 mg levodopa is equivalent to 300–400 mg levodopa in ordinary release or dispersible preparations. Hence the dose may need to be adjusted according to response
Phenytoin	90 mg phenytoin liquid is approximately equivalent to 100 mg phenytoin sodium capsules. Higher doses may be needed when administering liquid enterally, due to interactions
All 'retard' formulations	Total daily dose may need to be given more frequently

IRENE'S CASE

If Irene's swallowing function deteriorates she may need to have a radiologically inserted percutaneous gastrostomy tube, which is a safer technique for people with breathing problems. After insertion, nurses would need to contact the pharmacist to check how her medication preparations may need to be modified. Also in the initial stages, while she is adapting to this form of feeding, nurses would need to work closely with the dietician in evaluating her responses to feed preparations. In addition, if she has no oral intake, nurses need to plan with her tactics to ensure her oral hygiene and, if necessary, management of secretions. For Irene, the decision to initiate oral feeding may come at a time when she is facing serious end-of-life issues. It is outside the scope of this book to consider these issues but they are touched on in Chapter 14.

PROFESSIONAL AND ETHICAL ISSUES OF INITIATING AND WITHDRAWING NUTRITIONAL SUPPORT

If nurses act in accordance with the Nursing and Midwifery Council code of conduct then there should be no omission that renders the patient vulnerable to malnutrition, asphyxiation, aspiration pneumonia or dehydration because of their neurological impairment. There may be a time, however, in caring for some patients when the question of the patient's best interests about continuing enteral nutritional support may be raised by the patient, family or the professional care team. The ethical issues that arise and professional responsibilities are discussed further in Chapter 14.

SUMMARY

❏ Eating behaviours and diet are strongly associated with individual habit, social and psychological factors, and holistic care needs to take these into account.
❏ Neurological patients may have malnutrition brought on insidiously by prolonged inadequate intake as well as in the acute stages of illness.
❏ Swallowing involves sensory and motor nerves and a voluntary and reflex action as food passes through the oral, pharyngeal and oesophageal phases.

❏ Nurses can carry out early bedside swallowing screens after suitable training, referring to a speech and language therapist if appropriate.

❏ Nutritional assessment, supported by guidelines and protocols, is an essential interdisciplinary activity.

❏ Nursing skills in assisting patients with oral intake include good feeding techniques, reasoned selection of feeding aids and equipment, ability to prepare food to the correct consistency, effective nutritional monitoring and mouth care plans.

❏ Enteral feeding choices need to be evidence based and involve close liaison with a dietician.

❏ A pharmacist should be consulted on the appropriateness of drug formulations administered enterally.

❏ Professional and ethical issues will arise at the initiation and withdrawal of artificial feeding.

REFERENCES

Adam, S. K. (1994) Aspects of current research in enteral nutrition in the critically ill. *Care of the Critically Ill* **10** (6), 246–51.

Anderton, A. (1995) Reducing bacterial contamination in enteral tube feeds. *British Journal of Nursing* **4** (7), 368–76.

Bastow, M. D., Rawlings, J. and Allison, S. P. (1985) Overnight gastric tube feeding. *Clinical Nutrition* **4**, 7–11.

Bryce Evans, W., White, G. L., Wood, S. D., Hood, S. B. and Bailey, M. B. (1998) Managing dysphagia: fundamentals of primary care, available at http://www.medscape.com/CPG/ClinReviews/1998/v08.n08/c0808.01.evans

Collier, J. (2004) Enteral feeding: an overview. Nutrition and Dietetics Discussion Forum, available at http://www.dietetics.co.uk/article-enteral-feeding.asp

Cerulliu, J. and Malone, M. (1999) Assessment of drug related problems in clinical nutrition patients. *Journal of Parenteral and Enteral Nutrition* **23**, 218–21.

CREST (2004) *Guidelines for the Management of Enteral Tube Feeding in Adults*. Clinical Resource Efficiency Support Team, Belfast.

Davies, S. (1999) Dysphagia in acute strokes. *Nursing Standard* **13**, 30.

Dorman, F. (2003) Nutrition in critical illness. *Anaesthesia and Critical Care*, 114–16.

Elia, M. (1998) Trends in HETF. *Clinical Nutrition Update* **3** (2), 5–7.

Elia, M., Cottee, S., Holden, C., Micklewright, A., Pennington, C. and Plant, J. (1994) *Enteral Nutrition in the Community Working Party*, Report. BAPEN, Redditch.

6109301271761666166666111

Ellull, J., Barer, D. and Fall, S. (1997) Improving detection and management of swallowing problems in acute stroke: a multicentre study. *Cerebrovascular Disease* **7** (Supplement 4), 18.

Havard, M. and Tiziani, A. (1994) *A Nursing Guide to Drugs*, 4th edn. Churchill Livingstone, Edinburgh.

Hickey, J. (1997) *The Clinical Practice of Neurological and Neurosurgical Nursing*. Lippincott, New York.

Jamieson, E. M., McCall, J. M. and Whyte, L. A. (2002) *Clinical Nursing Practices*, 4th edn. Churchill Livingstone, Edinburgh.

Joanna Briggs Institute (2000) Identification and nursing management of dysphagia in adults with neurological impairment. *Best Practice* **4** (2).

Kennedy, J. F. (1997) Enteral feeding for the critically ill patient. *Nursing Standard* **11** (33), 39–43.

Leary, T., Fletcher, S. and Fellows, I. (2000) Enteral nutrition. Part 2: Its early use and often. *Care of the Critically Ill* **16** (2), 50–2.

MAG (Malnutrition Advisory Group) (2003) *Malnutrition Universal Screening Tool*. BAPEN Redditch.

Mallett, J. and Dougherty, L. (2000) *Manual of Clinical Nursing Procedures*. Blackwell Science, Oxford.

Metheny, N. M. (1996) *Fluid and Electrolyte Balance: Nursing Considerations*, 3rd edn. Lippincott, Philadelphia.

Parker, T., Neale, G. and Cottee, S. (1996) Management of artificial nutrition in East Anglia: a community study. *Journal of the Royal College of Physicians* **30** (1), 27–32.

RCP (Royal College of Physicians) (1999) *National Clinical Guidelines for Stroke*. The Intercollegiate Working Party for Stroke, Royal College of Physicians, London.

RCP (Royal College of Physicians) (2002) *National Clinical Guidelines for Stroke: Update 2002*. The Intercollegiate Working Party for Stroke, Royal College of Physicians, London.

Royal College of Speech and Language Therapists and British Diabetic Association (2003) National Descriptors for Texture Modification in Adults, available at http://www.bda.com

Thompson, F. C., Naysmith, M. R. and Lindsay, A. (2000) Managing drug therapy in patients receiving enteral and parenteral nutrition. *Hospital Pharmacist* **7** (6), 155–64.

Wood, A., Hill, K., McKenna, E. and Wilson, E. (1997) Developing a multidisciplinary protocol for enteral feeding. *Nursing in Critical Care* **2** (3), 126–8.

Zainal, G. (1994) Nutrition of critically ill people. *Intensive and Critical Care Nursing* **3**, 165–70.

Eliminating

7

INTRODUCTION

In western society, the activity of elimination has become very discreet and the products disposed of and treated in technologically advanced but almost invisible ways. In addition, the developmental gain in voluntary control of elimination function is a source of great personal dignity, and loss of control in later life can be deeply embarrassing. The elimination problems commonly experienced by people who have neurological impairment may be directly related to damage to the nerves supplying the bladder or colon, or they may be caused by reduced mobility or cognition. Many of the general principles of managing elimination disturbance apply to neurological patients, but there are also specific interventions. These are based on a thorough assessment to determine the nature of the problem and the most effective means of managing the symptoms and retraining elimination patterns. One of the difficulties in grasping the nature of neurogenic bowel and bladder problems is the terminology used, and it is important to grasp the concepts behind this terminology.

This chapter focuses on how to meet the needs of patients with elimination problems that are caused by motor or sensory dysfunction or by perceptual or cognitive impairment. These aspects are frequently encountered in neurological patients, and nurses need core skills in differentiating between storage or voiding problems and planning appropriate interventions.

LEARNING OUTCOMES

❏ Describe normal patterns of bowel and bladder elimination.
❏ Understand how neurological disease can lead to incontinence that is caused by neurogenic bladder, autonomic dys-

reflexia or by disorders of perception and cognition, and how this can affect these normal patterns.

❏ Appreciate emotional and psychological effects that altered elimination function has on the person.

❏ Discuss a range of different assessment techniques, diagnostic investigations techniques and interventions to manage bladder, sphincter and continence problems that neurological patients may have.

❏ Discuss a range of different assessment techniques, diagnostic investigations and interventions to manage bowel problems such as constipation and incontinence that neurological patients may have.

❏ Discuss the role of the interdisciplinary team and specialist nurses in managing elimination needs.

STORAGE AND VOIDING OF URINE

Normal patterns of elimination

The urinary bladder is a hollow muscular bag that has a smooth muscle middle coat known as the *detrusor* muscle. This coat has *stretch receptors* that can detect when the muscle wall is distended by urine. During filling, the bladder wall is relaxed to accommodate a urine volume of up to about 500 ml. When the bladder is full, the stretch receptors are stimulated (see Figure 7.1). They conduct the message to the sacral region of the spinal cord. The voiding reflex then causes the bladder to contract, at the same time relaxing the external sphincter and thus allowing urine to be passed. In some patients, this mechanism is disturbed and the external sphincter does not relax at the same time as the detrusor muscle contracts (*detrusor–sphincter dyssynergia*). For people without continence problems, the voiding reflex can be controlled voluntarily by inhibitory messages from the motor cortex of the brain.

Dysfunctional bladder

The most common urinary problems that people with neurological diseases experience is with the *storage or emptying* of urine or even both. These problems occur with varying degrees of intensity and incontinence (see Box 7.1), and present a

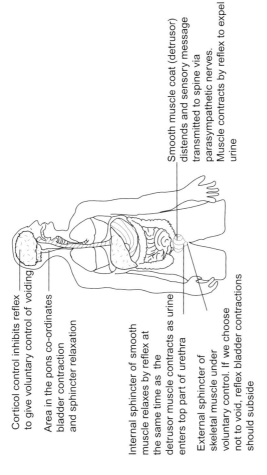

Corticol control inhibits reflex to give voluntary control of voiding

Area in the pons co-ordinates bladder contraction and sphincter relaxation

Internal sphincter of smooth muscle relaxes by reflex at the same time as the detrusor muscle contracts as urine enters top part of urethra

External sphincter of skeletal muscle under voluntary control. If we choose not to void, reflex bladder contractions should subside

Smooth muscle coat (detrusor) distends and sensory message transmitted to spine via parasympathetic nerves. Muscle contracts by reflex to expel urine

Figure 7.1 Muscle actions in micturition.

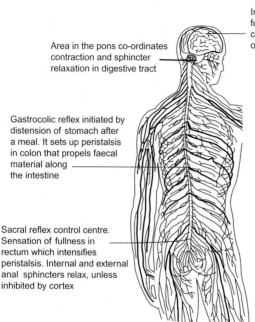

Integration of sense of fullness in rectum with motor cortex gives voluntary control of anal sphincter

Area in the pons co-ordinates contraction and sphincter relaxation in digestive tract

Gastrocolic reflex initiated by distension of stomach after a meal. It sets up peristalsis in colon that propels faecal material along the intestine

Sacral reflex control centre. Sensation of fullness in rectum which intensifies peristalsis. Internal and external anal sphincters relax, unless inhibited by cortex

Figure 7.2 Nerve and muscle control in bowel evacuation.

Box 7.1 Classification of urinary incontinence (Hickey 1997)

- *Urge incontinence.* Diagnosed by urodynamic investigation. Also called detrusor hyperreflexia.
- *Stress incontinence.* Observed urine loss when there is an increase in abdominal pressure, overdistended bladder or absence of dextrose contraction.
- *Overflow.* May present in different ways, e.g. constant dribbling, urge or stress symptoms. May be due to underactive detrusor or to outlet obstruction.
- *Loss of inhibition by cortex.* Voluntary control is lost and bladder voids spontaneously.

---

constant risk of urinary tract infection. The vocabulary to describe bladder dysfunctions may differ in different textbooks, particularly American textbooks. In the UK, the term *neurogenic bladder* is used to describe problems of bladder storage or voiding that are caused by impaired nerve function. Different types of neurogenic bladder are listed in Table 7.1.

NURSING ASSESSMENT

The aim of nursing assessment is to identify the physiological nature of the problem and the impact it has on the patient's social and psychological attitude to life. There may be specialist nurses who can help from either a neurologically specific condition, such as multiple sclerosis nurse specialist, or stroke care nurse, or from a more general perspective such as a generic continence advisor. Following this, a thorough discussion with the patient on the intervention options and ways of evaluating their effectiveness can help evolve a satisfactory management programme for the individual (Bardsley 2000; Griffith 2002).

Aspects to assess include the following:

- The frequency, amount and timing of passing urine? Is nocturia a problem?
- Does this indicate whether the problem is primarily of storage, voiding or dyssynergia?
- Is there incomplete emptying? Is there post-micturition residual urine greater than 100 ml? This can be assessed by abdominal ultrasound of the bladder or by intermittent catheterisation. If more than 100 ml, it may cause frequency and urgency (Woodward 2004).
- Is there a total inability to void?
- Are there recurrent urinary tract infections? Is there pain on passing urine or other signs of urinary infection?
- Is there urge incontinence or overflow incontinence (see Box 7.1)?
- A diary can help to collect data and ensure reliability over time about the patterns emerging of frequency, amount and timing.
- The diary can correlate fluid intake and record episodes of incontinence (Hickey 1997; Schwarz 2001; Griffith 2002).

- Is there any evidence of dribbling, urge or stress incontinence that may indicate overflow from an incompletely emptied bladder?
- Is the person able to delay voiding?
- Does the person have sensation of fullness in the bladder?
- Is the bladder distended?
- Are there other factors which may affect continence, e.g. cognitive or sensory deficits, depression?
- Is the person taking any medication that can affect urine output (sedatives, diuretics, alpha-adrenergic drugs that can affect sphincter tone, or calcium channel blockers that can reduce smooth muscle contractility causing retention with overflow, anticholinergics)?
- Are there any environmental factors or mobility factors that affect continence?
- Is the problem primarily motor, sensory or cognitive, or a combination of these factors?
- Does the person need specialist assessment or further urodynamic investigations? These can help to identify flow rate and residual urine and to differentiate between detrusor dyssynergia and stress incontinence.

INTERVENTION OPTIONS

Following assessment, an individual plan of care is developed with the patient, which may include the following interventions.

Bladder retraining

The aim of treatment here is to decrease or eliminate episodes of incontinence, as the patient gradually increases the time between voiding until a normal 3–4 hourly interval is achieved. Bladder retraining can be effective in treating urinary frequency and urge incontinence, and be an effective alternative to drug therapy (Weiss 1991; Anders 1999). Patients need to be carefully selected, as motivation needs to be high and patients ideally need to be ambulant and cognitively aware (Woodward 2004). Although bladder training is currently recommended practice for an overactive bladder, Wallace *et al.* (2004) concluded that the limited evidence available renders conclusions about its

Table 7.1 Types of neurogenic bladder.

	Effects of impairment	Cause	Possible intervention
Detrusor hyperreflexia	Reduced bladder capacity Urgency Frequency Nocturia Urge incontinence	Messages from the brain are not inhibiting the voiding reflex and the bladder is overactive Common in multiple sclerosis, stroke, brain injury	Scheduled voiding Condom-type catheter Drugs such as oxybutinin (Bardsley 1999; Schwarz 2001)
Detrusor sphincter dyssynergia	Incomplete emptying of the bladder with large amounts of residual urine. Interrupted flow	Damage in brain stem where detrusor muscle and sphincter muscle activity is co-ordinated	Reflex-triggering techniques Intermittent catherisation Drugs (Woodward 2004)
Detrusor arreflexia	Increased bladder capacity, high residual urine, involuntary voiding, overflow incontinence, frequency, urgency, recurrent infections	Impairment in lower motor neurones causing weakened bladder muscle contraction and reduced sensation of fullness	Intermittent catherisation Valsalva's manoeuvre Crede's method (Hickey 1997)
Mixed	Some patients may experience discomfort associated with more than one type of neurogenic bladder		

effectiveness tentative and that definitive research has yet to be conducted.

A bladder-retraining programme educates the patient in the pathophysiology and the techniques of resisting or inhibiting the sense of urgency, delaying voiding and scheduling voiding. The fluid intake can also be manipulated to help regulate the bladder and facilitate the storage and passage of larger volumes of urine less frequently.

Habit training
Habit training aims to keep the patient dry by asking them to empty the bladder at regular intervals, trying to match this as much as possible with the patient's regular habit. Patients are not usually suitable for bladder training by asking them to delay voiding or by resisting the urge to pass water (Hickey 1997).

Prompted voiding
Prompted voiding for cognitively impaired people attempts to increase their awareness of the sensation of bladder fullness and their awareness that incontinence has occurred. Praise is used to reinforce episodes of continence. Brain-injured patients will need a sustained programme that helps them with orientation to the environment, clues to prompt topographical memory and habit training every two or three hours. Success in voiding or not must be recorded since this can indicate a problem with incomplete emptying which will need to be assessed and treated.

Pelvic floor muscle training exercises
Pelvic floor muscle training exercises can help, although persistence and conscientiousness are needed to bring about results. The perivaginal muscles and anal sphincter are drawn in, held for a count of ten, and then relaxed for a count of ten. About 50–100 of these need to be done each day for four to six weeks to notice any improvement (Hickey 1997). Pelvic floor exercises can also be asssisted by biofeedback under supervision of a physiotherapist. Electrodes are placed on the abdominal wall and external sphincter. Nerve signals are routed through a monitor and the activity of the pelvic floor muscles are displayed visually.

Suprabladder compression to elicit reflex
Valsava's manoeuvre is used to create suprapubic bladder compression, using palm pressure to assist in emptying the atonic bladder.

Bladder triggering techniques
These techniques stimulate the sacro-lumbar dermatomes to increase sensory input. The suprapubic area is manually tapped, pubic hairs pulled or the inside of the thighs stroked.

Bladder-stimulating vibration
Bladder-stimulating vibration is carried out using a hand-held device called the Queen Square bladder stimulator. The vibrating stimulus to the suprapubic region when the person is sitting on the toilet can significantly improve urinary symptoms in people with neurogenic bladder (Dasgupta *et al.* 1997), and can help start micturition, improve flow and reduce the residual volume.

Intermittent catheterisation
Intermittent catheterisation is recommended for patients with incomplete bladder emptying and post-micturition volume above 100 ml (Clanet and Brassett 2000), since treatment is less successful in the presence of high residual volumes (Dasgupta and Fowler 2002). The frequency of clean intermittent catheterisation depends on the individual need of the patient and on whether they do this themselves or whether someone does it for them. Most people with sufficient determination can master the technique. The fear of introducing infection is common, but as long as a clean technique is used, the overall effect can be to reduce infection since stagnant urine is not allowed to accumulate (Woodward 1995, 1996; MST 2000; Woodward and Rew 2003).

Winder (2002) offers general guidance:

- When planning the number of times a patient needs to catheterise, the urinary volumes plus residual volumes should not be greater than 500 ml at each catheterisation. Most people aim for two to three times a day and before bed if nocturia is a problem (MST 2000).

- If a patient does not empty the bladder, the total bladder capacity should not exceed 500 ml between catheterisations. It is not advisable to exceed a residual of 100 ml between catheterisations as this may cause urine infections.
- More frequent catheterisation or anticholinergic medication may help if a patient is wet between catheterisations.

Pharmacological interventions

Anticholinergic medications inhibit the action of acetylcholine to stimulate the bladder. This reduces the contractions of the overactive detrusor muscle. Such medications include oxybutin or tolterodine. Of these, tolterodine has been shown in one study (Abrams 1998) to be as effective and better tolerated than oxybutinin. O'Leary *et al.* (2003), however, found that slow-release oxybutinin was safe and effective in patients with detrusor hyperreflexia secondary to spinal cord injury. Some patients may find the side effects of oxybutinin, such as dry mouth or constipation, troublesome and these may be minimised by adjusting the dose, frequency or switching to a controlled-release preparation (Woodward 2004). Also, artificial saliva in spray or tablet form may be prescribed if bladder control is good but mouth dryness unpleasant. Anticholinergic medication can also impair the ability of the bladder to empty properly, which can be managed by an intermittent catheterisation programme.

It seems that Louise (see case study in the section on How to Use this Book) has an areflexic bladder. This can be confirmed by palpating the bladder and using a bladder scanner post-voiding to see if the residual volume is greater than 100 ml. If a scanner is not available, a urethral catheter can be inserted measure residual volume. Initially this urethral catheter can be fitted with a flip-flow valve to ensure that Louise does not go into retention. As the steroids reduce inflammation, the catheter may be replaced by other bladder retraining techniques, such as applying pressure over the bladder or by standing up, turning round and sitting down and trying again after an initial voiding has been made. However, the steroid therapy may improve motor function more than sensory function for Louise, which may present her with more problems in the future.

Bladder function can also be disturbed by constipation. Two litres of fluid a day, preferably without caffeine, may help for bulk, as will a healthy diet with soluble and insoluble fibre, and laxative if necessary.

While Louise has an underactive bladder at the moment, there may be times when she suffers, in common with many people who suffer from multiple sclerosis, an overactive or hyperreflexive bladder or detrusor hyperreflexia. If this happens, then bladder retraining and oral anticholinergic medication as outlined in the section on bladder retraining will help the symptoms of urgency and frequency. For those who experience urgency, frequency and have difficulty emptying completely, the best combination is oral anticholinergic medication and regular intermittent catheterisation (MST 2000).

Bedwetting and nocturia can be a problem, interfering with sleep, increasing fatigue and contributing to pressure sore risk. Desmopressin reduces the amount of urine produced by the kidneys and its action can last 3–6 hours. It can be useful for patients to take before going to sleep and who do not respond to anticholinergics alone (Dasgupta and Fowler 2002), and can be taken as a spray or in tablet form in the evening together with controlled fluid intake. There is a slight risk of hyponatraemia, and for this reason serum sodium levels should be monitored. (Dasgupta and Fowler 2003)

OTHER PROBLEMS CAUSED BY NEUROGENIC BLADDER IMPAIRMENT

Autonomic dysreflexia is a serious complication of spinal cord injury or damage above cord level at the thoracic vertebrae T6 to T8. Autonomic dysreflexia can arise if bladder and bowel elimination are not properly managed. The reflex that bladder or bowel fullness generates is disordered and an uncontrolled disturbance of autonomic function develops that dangerously deranges homeostasis.

The symptoms are:

- sudden rise in blood pressure
- slowing pulse

- sweating
- severe headache
- gooseflesh

Treatment should be immediate, as follows:

- Place patient in sitting position to reduce blood pressure.
- Monitor blood pressure and other vital signs.
- Drain urinary bladder safely by catheterisation or check that catheter is not kinked or blocked.
- Check rectum for impaction of faeces.
- Remove other potential triggers that may cause nociceptive impulses to the spinal cord.
- Obtain urine specimen for culture and sensitivity.
- Administer medication prescribed to reduce blood pressure.
- Educate patient about complications and actions to prevent and alleviate it (Hickey 1997).

URINARY COLLECTING AND STORING DEVICES

As the management of elimination problems evolves, it may be necessary to use a collecting device or padding. For stress incontinence there are several devices, such as condom-style sheath, that may be fitted over the urethral meatus. These use suction or adhesive to stay in place or absorbent padding may be used.

Longer-term management of emptying problems may need long-term catheterisation (Brosnall *et al.* 2004; Jamieson *et al.* 2004). Although all current guidelines suggest that long-term catheterisation should be a last resort (Jamieson *et al.* 2002; Mallett and Doughterty 2000), many patients have long-term neurological problems and find that urethral or suprapubic catheterisation meets their needs (Peate 1997). The relative advantages and disadvantages of the suprapubic mode are set out in Table 7.2.

As with a urethral catheter, the collecting device can be free drainage into a bag or regulated through a catheter valve. The valve ensures that urine is stored in the bladder and is then emptied through the catheter straight into the toilet or bag. A spare catheter should always be to hand, since if it comes out it should be replaced within 20 minutes, otherwise the opening will close. Very often patients can be taught to do this

Table 7.2 Advantages and disadvantages of suprapubic catheters for managing long-term incontinence (Addison and Mould 2000, with permission).

Advantages	Disadvantages
Less trauma to urethra caused by catheterisation	Bowel perforation/haemorrhage at cystotomy formation
Reduced urethral stricture rate	Cystotomy complications
Safer to perform when pelvic trauma is present	
Voiding assessment is easier	Some patients experience pain/discomfort/irritation
Long-term catheterisation	Some dislike altered body image
Less infection to the urinary tract	Possible long-term risk of squamous cell carcinoma
Less difficulty with sexual intercourse	Urethral leakage, particularly in females
Less pain/discomfort	Bladder stones

themselves. The catheter should not be replaced if trauma has been caused and the area is bleeding.

Bladder washouts

Catheters may be become blocked by detrusor spasm, twisted drainage tubing, or constipation. The usual reason, however, is encrustation on the catheter surface and within its lumen (Getliffe 1996; Mallet and Dougherty 2000). There is little evidence, however, to support the notion of routine bladder washouts to prevent encrustations and blockage and further work needs to identify whether regular washouts might adversely affect the bladder wall because of the acidity of the solutions. Getliffe (1994) suggests 'mini-washouts' using volumes of 10–20 ml of normal saline, which would be sufficient to irrigate the lumen and catheter tip without inducing bladder irritation. If a blockage already exists, this may be mechanically dislodged by 'milking' the tube before replacing the catheter or by irrigation with an appropriate fluid such as the Suby range.

Bladder dysfunction and incontinence can be very disabling and have many adverse consequences (NICE 2003), including great emotional distress, curtailed social activities, psychosexual disturbance, disturbed sleep and loss of self-esteem. The

NICE guidelines make several recommendations, noting that many of the issues are not specific to people with multiple sclerosis and are similar to those faced by other people with a neurogenic bladder or neurological problems that compromise continence. The guidelines that cover the main issues discussed in this chapter include:

- detection and diagnosis of disturbed bladder physiology;
- management of disrupted bladder function;
- diagnosis and treatment of urinary tract infections;
- management of intractable incontinence;

A summary of the main likely bladder and continence problems suffered by people with different neurological conditions is shown in Table 7.3.

Ella (see case study in the section on How to Use this Book) is incontinent of urine, a situation that may well be adding to her distress. Her nurse should ensure that any episodes of incontinence are dealt with quickly with the minimum of fuss and carry out a full assessment as outlined to try to establish if there is a pattern to her urinary elimination. The assessment may indicate whether Ella has an inhibited bladder, incomplete bladder emptying, or retention or urge problems. A continence chart and fluid balance chart should be maintained to observe if there is a pattern to her incontinence. Ella should be given reassurance that this may only be a temporary problem until she becomes more mobile. Pads could be used initially, with close monitoring of Ella's skin integrity. The problem could be closely linked to Ella's altered communication, as she may be embarrassed to call out to nursing staff or may be unable to understand the nurse call system. The information gathered in the communication assessment and an understanding of any perceptual or cognitive problems can be used to help her develop effective strategies to communicate her elimination needs.

BOWEL STORAGE AND EVACUATION

Movements of the large intestine

Neural control of digestion and bowel evacuation occurs at different levels of the nervous system, similar to the levels of

Table 7.3 Urinary continence problems people with neurological problems may develop.

	Altered sensation	Altered motor ability	Altered perception cognition	Possible problems
Stroke	Lost sensation of bladder fullness Lost sensation of being wet	Hemiplegia limiting movement and activity, detrusor hyperreflexia, external sphincter dyssenergia	Receptive or expressive aphasia	Urge incontinence, incomplete bladder emptying, urine retention
Multiple sclerosis	Of passing urine, sense of wetness	Detrusor–sphincter disturbance Mobility may worsen at same time as bladder problems Spasticity		Diminished bladder capacity, reduced flow rate, incomplete emptying, interrupted stream, urgency, nocturia
Parkinson's disease	Autonomic disturbance	Autonomic disturbance Slow to initiate movement On–off phases 'Freezing' Choreiform movement Drop in blood pressure on standing	Hallucination Delusion	Frequency, urgency retention. Often because of anticholinergic drugs
Dementia, acquired brain injury	Disturbed sensory pathways, Reduced awareness	Spasticity Paralysis Posture	Aphasia Confusion Agitation	Uninhibited neurogenic bladder, urgency frequency, inability to suppress voiding urge, unawareness of voiding urge

bladder elimination. These include the cortical and sub-cortical levels and the spinal cord, ending in the sacral reflex at S2, S3 and S4 (see Figure 7.2, p. 156). The autonomic nerves at different levels in the body initiate peristaltic movement, although normal development allows conscious control of the anal sphincters. The parasympathetic nerves cause contraction of the gut wall (peristalsis) that move faeces along the colon and to the rectum. When the wall of the rectum is distended, the sensation is conducted by the sacral nerves (S2, S3 and S4) to the spinal cord. A reflex then relaxes the internal and external anal sphincters to allow defecation.

The primary muscles of defecation are therefore the abdominal muscles, the diaphragm and the levator muscles of the anal canal. They work together to increase an abdominal pressure that aid in expelling the contents. The ways in which neurological impairments can affect bowel function are shown in Box 7.2.

NURSING ASSESSMENT

Nursing assessment needs to establish the nature of the bowel problem and to develop care plan interventions that identify a clear goal. The care plan may involve ongoing management of bowel dysfunction that is unlikely to improve. With other patients, the goal may be to return to continence over time or to establish a regular bowel habit. Generally, however, for most people the overall aim is to eliminate a soft, formed stool every 1–3 days.

Aspects to consider in assessment include the following:

- What is the bowel elimination pattern? What is the frequency, the characteristics of the stool? The Bristol stool form chart can be used for reliability in estimating consistency.
- Does the patient show any signs of discomfort or straining? Is there a record of the previous bowel pattern?
- Is there any abdominal distension or discomfort?
- Is there any loss of appetite or swallowing impairment?
- What other risk factors are there? Is there any risk that autonomic dysreflexia could develop from bowel distension?
- Is there evidence of fibre and fluid intake over the preceding 7 days?

- Is the person incontinent of faeces? Is this related to damage at the cortical level or at the spinal level? Is the incontinence related to pelvic floor weakness or sphincter incompetence?
- Is the patient on any drugs with the side effect of constipation or diarrhoea? The following groups of drugs are associated with constipation: anticholinergics, anticonvulsants, antidepressants, any Parkinson drugs, antipsychotics, calcium supplements, diuretics, iron tablets, opiates (MST 2000).
- What was the patient's normal bowel pattern before illness? How is it managed if it is an ongoing problem?
- Does the patient have brain injury that might prevent the sensation of rectal fullness or awareness of spontaneous evacuation?

Box 7.2 Potential problems caused by neurological disease

- *Brain injury* voluntary control of defecation may be lost because the sensation of rectal fullness is not transmitted to the brain, and the spinal reflex evacuates the bowel spontaneously. This type of dysfunction is called *uninhibited neurogenic bowel.*
- *Dementia, multiple sclerosis, spinal cord injury or cerebral tumours* may also impair a person's ability to sense or perceive rectal fullness (Hickey 1997; Schwarz 2001).
- Bowel problems may also accompany neurological disease because of:
  - altered muscle tone in abdomen, colon and sphincter muscles causing spasticity or flaccidity;
  - low activity levels;
  - delayed gastric emptying;
  - reduced intestinal peristalsis;
  - side effects of drug treatments used;
  - swallowing problems leading to inadequate mastication or nutrition;
  - inadequate fluid intake;
  - problems with intolerance of enteral feeding preparations.

INTERVENTIONS

Bowel retraining and management of incontinence depend on the extent of neural damage and cognitive abilities. However, in the short term the goal is to establish a pattern of elimination, taking into account that the patient may also have problems with attention, memory, concentration or communication.

Disappointingly, Coggrave *et al.* (2004) concluded from their systematic review that no evidence-based recommendations could be made for bowel care in people with neurological diseases. The main result of their study showed that psyllium was associated with increased stool frequency in people with Parkinson's disease but not altered colonic transit time. Some rectal preparations to initiate defecation produced faster results than others and that different time schedules for administration of rectal medication may produce different bowel responses. One trial also showed that manual evacuation might be more effective than oral or rectal administration (Addison and Smith 2000). In addition, the study concluded that cisapride does not seem to have clinically useful effects in people with spinal cord injury. It has in fact has been withdrawn in some countries because it can provoke rare but dangerous arrhythmias and high reflex contractions in hyperactive spinal cord injured bladders (Coggrave *et al.* 2004).

The general recommendations from this systematic review suggest dietary counselling, taking into account personal goals, life schedules and obligations of the individual. A bowel retraining programme, together with appropriate medications that promote or inhibit bowel function should be established on a trial-and-error basis and regularly evaluated.

The following principles have been shown to be effective in a bowel retraining programme (Hickey 1997; Schwarz 2001):

- Before beginning a training programme, make sure the lower bowel is empty (use an enema if necessary).
- Agree a time of day for a bowel movement and a regular eating pattern.
- Agree a high-fibre diet that is to the patient's liking and use a bulking agent if necessary.

- Ensure a fluid intake of between 2 and 2.5 litres per day, unless there is a fluid restriction.
- Insert a suppository on the first day. The purpose of this is to increase rectal sensation and to stimulate the ano-rectal reflex and thus awareness of the urge to defecate. It also stimulates lubrication of the intestinal tract.
- Repeat suppository insertion on the second day at the same time. If it is effective, repeat the insertion every other day, although some patients may still need it every day. Once a routine is established, the suppositories can be discontinued.
- If possible, the patient should be seated on the commode or toilet to allow privacy. Increase intra-abdominal pressure and allow gravity to assist defecation. The correct posture, bracing the abdomen and bulging to increase abdominal pressure may all assist the passage of stool from the sigmoid colon into the rectum.
- Biofeedback or sphincter and pelvic floor exercises may have some therapeutic effect but the evidence is limited (Norton *et al.* 2002). Exercises to strengthen the abdominal muscles and diaphragm can also help strengthen peristalsis and defecation where constipation, slow transit or low intra-abdominal pressure is a problem.
- Administer medications to modify the stool consistency or reduce the frequency of bowel movements. The main categories of laxatives and their actions are shown in Table 7.4.
- Collaborate with other health team members to individualise bowel care programme. The team may include the dietician, physiotherapist or specialist nurses in neurology or continence management.
- The occasional use of anal continence plugs may help to control faecal incontinence and prevent loss of stool at an embarrassing time. It is a sponge foam plug with a gauze strip for removal. On contact with the rectal mucosa, the plug opens up to form a seal.

PSYCHOSOCIAL EFFECTS
Problems with bladder and bowel dysfunction may have an impact on a patient's emotional well-being, social life and

Table 7.4 Categories and actions of laxatives.

	Action	Side effects	Examples
Bulking agents	Hydrophilic action so that gut absorbs water and stimulates peristalsis, effective in 12–24 hours	May cause flatulence Obstruction or impaction if insufficient water is drunk	Normacol, Fybogel (ispaghula)
Osmotic laxative	Stimulate peristalsis by exerting local effect on the gut wall causing slight irritation, bulking and increased peristalsis	Flatulence and abdominal cramps, diarrhoea	Lactulose Sodium phosphate enema
Stimulant laxatives	Increased secretion of water and electrolytes in colon, increased peristalsis	Abdominal cramps or colic, diarrhoea, severe purgation	Bisacodyl, senna, glycerin suppositories
Emollient laxative	Softens faeces by decreasing surface tension allowing defecation without straining	Abdominal cramps and colic, diarrhoea	Docusate sodium Microlax enema

sexual relationship or functioning. The main principles of care have been outlined in this chapter, but making contact with the many support groups incorporated in the neurological alliance can not only help nurse, patients and relatives with practical tips on managing dysfunction but also give emotional and psychological support.

CASES

Anwah
Will she be managed with pads and frequent changes? Observe consistency of stool and ensure good hydration.

Joyce
Is spasticity interfering with posture and position for elimination or making self-cleaning difficult?

Fred
Fred, in common with other Parkinson's disease sufferers, could
have frequency and urgency of his urine output and chronic
constipation, caused by anti-Parkinson drugs, slowed gut moti-
lity, immobility and dehydration. After assessment, nurses need
to select the appropriate interventions as outlined in the chapter.

Irene
Because the lower motor neurones are affected, Irene may have
underactive bladder function and constipation as a result of
muscle weakness and dysfunctional innervation of the bowel.

SUMMARY
❏ Neurogenic bladder problems cause storage and voiding
problems.
❏ The three main types of neurogenic bladder are detrusor
hyperreflexia, detrusor sphincter dyssynergia and detrusor
arreflexia. Each gives rise to different problems.
❏ The main intervention options depend on whether the
problem is with storage or voiding and include bladder
training, bladder stimulation, pelvic floor exercises, drug
treatment, intermittent catherisation or urethral or suprapubic catheterisation.
❏ The risk of autonomic dysreflexia with uncontrolled homeostasis increases with mismanaged bladder and bowel elimination.
❏ Bowel elimination difficulties may be caused by lack of
mobility, inadequate oral intake, loss of sensation, impaired
muscle tone, loss of voluntary control, communication problems or cognitive deficits.
❏ A bowel-retraining programme can be helpful in gaining
some control or predictability of bowel evacuation.
❏ Laxatives may be used but need to be carefully selected
based on assessment of the problem.

REFERENCES
Abrams, P., Freeman, R., Anderstrom, C. and Mattiason, A. (1998)
Tolterodine, a new antimuscarinic agent, as effective but better
tolerated than oxybutinin in patients with an overactive bladder.
British Journal of Urology **81**, 801–10.

Addison, R. and Mould, C. (2000) Risk assessment in suprapubic catheterization. *Nursing Standard* **14** (36), 43–6.

Addison, R. and Smith, M. (2000) Digital Rectal Examination and Manual Removal of Faeces: Guidance for Nurses. Royal College of Nursing, London.

Anders, K. (1999) Bladder retraining. *Professional Nurse* **14**, 334–6.

Bardsley, A. (1999) A sense of control. *Nursing Times* **95**, 31.

Bardsley, A. (2000) The neurogenic bladder. *Nursing Standard* **14** (22), 39–41.

Brosnall, J., Jull, A. and Tracy, C. (2004) Types of urethral catheters for management of short term voiding problems in hospitalised adults (Cochrane Review). In *The Cochrane Library*, Issue 3. John Wiley, Chichester.

Clanet, M. G. and Brassett, D. (2000) The management of multiple sclerosis patients. *Current Opinion in Neurology* **13**, 263–70.

Coggrave, M., Wiesel, P. H., Norton, C. and Brazelli, M. (2004) Management of faecal incontinence and constipation in adults with central neurological disease (Cochrane Review). In *The Cochrane Library*, Issue 3. John Wiley, Chichester.

Dasgupta, R. and Fowler, C. J. (2002) Sexual and urological dysfunction in multiple sclerosis: better understanding and improved therapies. *Current Opinion in Neurology* **15**, 271–8.

Dasgupta, R. and Fowler, C. J. (2003) Bladder bowel and sexual dysfunction in multiple sclerosis. *Drugs* **63**(2), 153–66.

Dasgupta, R., Haslam, C., Goodwin, R. and Fowler, C. J. (1997) The Queen Square bladder stimulator: a device for assisting emptying of the neurogenic bladder. *British Journal of Urology* **80**, 234–7.

Getliffe, K. and Dolmnan, M. (1997) *Promoting Continence: A Clinical Research Resource*. Baillière Tindall, London.

Getliffe, K. A. (1994) The use of bladder washouts to to reduce urinary catheter encrustations. *British Journal of Urology* **73**, 696–700.

Getliffe, K. A. (1996) Bladder instillations and bladder washouts in the management of catheterised patients. *Journal of Advanced Nursing* **23**, 548–54.

Griffith, G. (2002) Importance of continence advice for people with multiple sclerosis. *British Journal of Nursing* **11** (21), 1363–71.

Hickey, J. (1997) *The Clinical Practice of Neurological and Neurosurgical Nursing*, 4th edn. Lippincott, New York.

Jamieson, E. M., McCall, J. M. and Whyte, L. A. (2002) *Clinical Nursing Practices*, 4th edn, Churchill Livingstone, Edinburgh.

Jamieson, J., Maguire, S. and McCann, J. (2004) Catheter policies for management of long term voiding problems in adults with neurogenic bladder disorders (Cochrane Review). In *The Cochrane Library*, Issue 3. John Wiley, Chichester.

Mallett, J. and Dougherty, L. (2000) *Manual of Clinical Nursing Procedures*, 5th edn. Blackwell Science, Oxford.

MST (Multiple Sclerosis Trust) (2000) *Multiple Sclerosis Information for Health and Social Care Professionals*. Multiple Sclerosis Trust, Letchworth.

NICE (2003) *Multiple Sclerosis: National Clinical Guidelines for Diagnosis and Management in Primary and Secondary Care*. National Institute for Clinical Excellence/National Collaborating Centre for Chronic Conditions, London.

Norton, C., Hosker, G. and Brazelli, M. (2002) Biofeedback and/or sphincter exercises for the treatment of faecal incontinence (Cochrane Review). In *The Cochrane Library*, Issue 3. John Wiley, Chichester.

O'Leary, M., Erickson, J. R., Smith, C. P., McDermott, C., Horton, J. and Chancellor, M. B. (2003) Effect of controlled release oxybutinin on neurogenic bladder function in spinal cord injury. *Journal of Spinal Cord Medicine* **26** (2), 159–62.

Peate, I. (1997) Patient management following suprapubic catheterisation. *British Journal of Nursing* **6** (10), 555–62.

Schwarz, R. R. (2001) Alterations in bladder elimination. In: Stewart-Amadei, C. and Kinkel, J. A. (eds), *AANN's Neuroscience Nursing: Human Response to Neurologic Dysfunction*. W.B. Saunders, New York, chapter 27.

Wallace, S. A., Roe, B., Williams, K. and Palmer, M. (2004) Bladder training for urinary incontinence in adults (Cochrane Review). In *The Cochrane Library*, Issue 3. John Wiley, Chichester.

Weiss, B. D. (1991) Nonpharmacologic treatment of urinary incontinence. *American Family Physician* **44** (2), 579–86.

Winder, A. (2002) Intermittent self catheterisation. *Nursing Times* **98** (48), 50–1.

Woodward, S. (1995) Assessment of urinary incontinence in neuroscience patients. *British Journal of Nursing* **4**, 254–8.

Woodward, S. (1996) Impact of neurological problems on urinary incontinence. *British Journal of Nursing* **5**, 906–13.

Woodward, S. (2004) Current management of neurogenic bladder in patients with MS. *British Journal of Nursing* **13** (7), 362–70.

Woodward, S. and Rew, M. (2003) Patients quality of life and clean intermittent self-catheterisation. *British Journal of Nursing* **12**, 1066–74.

8 | Washing and Dressing

INTRODUCTION

Self-care activities such as washing oneself, brushing teeth and hair and applying products such as deodorant or scents to enhance social acceptance are perceived as fundamental social skills. Dressing oneself and choice of clothing are also an expression of individuality as well as a way of conforming to social norms. Neurological impairments affect a person's self-care abilities not only physically in a number of different ways but can also have an effect on the way people see themselves and other people see them. People with a neurological impairment have different dependency levels, and some may alter from day to day or even hour to hour. Many people can be completely independent in this activity if provided with the right equipment and environment. A sensitive approach to levels of independence is extremely important, since personal hygiene is part of a person's identity and the way that one dresses is closely linked with the sense of one's social self, self-esteem and self-image.

While it is a clear nursing responsibility to maintain a good level of hygiene and grooming for patients, these need to be negotiated as carefully as possible to ensure that safety and well-being are maintained, while autonomy is respected and individuality acknowledged.

The aim of this chapter is to identify the neurological deficits that can handicap a person in realising their wishes with regard to their personal hygiene and presentation of self, and the ways in which nurses can help people overcome these deficits.

LEARNING OBJECTIVES

❏ Outline the range of neurological impairments that can affect independence in washing, dressing and grooming and appreciate the effect this has on a person's sense of social belonging

❏ Describe a range of aids and equipment that can facilitate washing and dressing activities

❏ Discuss a range of strategies, techniques and nursing interventions that can maintain personal hygiene standards, foster independence and minimise fatigue in neurological patients.

DEFICITS THAT MAY CAUSE PROBLEMS

Neurological impairments that arise from a range of neurological conditions need to be carefully assessed for the effect on independence in the activities of washing and dressing.

• *Motor problems* may cause weakness, co-ordination problems, paralysis, spasticity, contractions, reduced range of joint movement, impaired grip, inability to walk unaided, poor sitting balance.

• *Sensory problems* may render patients unable to detect water temperature or to recognise when garments are chafing, wrinkled or causing irritation.

• *Perceptual problems* that include *agnosia*, where the ability to recognise familiar objects is impaired. It may be difficult to find items such as soap, flannel or toothbrush. Perceptual problems also include a movement planning problem, *apraxia*, where the patient has difficulty planning and organising movements.

• *Body image deficit*, the lack of visual and mental image of one's body or body scheme deficit, or difficulty in perceiving the position of the body and the relationship of body parts. This can cause confusion over the sides of the body, difficulty understanding left and right, neglect of the affected side of the body or the environment, and failure to recognise or denial of the deficit and dexterity problems (Edmans *et al.* 2001).

• *Spatial relations deficit* may cause *figure–ground deficit*, where the person may be unable to distinguish a towel from bed linen, or find a brush in a cluttered draw; *form constancy deficit*, where a person may have difficulty discriminating between a water jug and a flower vase; difficulty in following concepts such as in/out, in front of/behind, up/down. Patients may find it difficult to find the shampoo behind the wash bag.

- *Topographical disorientation* may mean that patients have difficulty finding the way to the bathroom.
- *Depth and distance deficit* where the patient has difficulty in judging these and may not recognise when the wash basin, bath or tooth mug is full.
- *Cognitive problems* may follow from problems with attention, memory, classifying and organising information to enable reasoning, and from executive deficits in self-awareness, goal setting, self-monitoring and self-evaluation.

All or any of these can impair a patient's independence in self-care. The potential deficits in a range of neurological conditions is shown in Table 8.1.

COMMON PRACTICAL DIFFICULTIES IN WASHING AND DRESSING

Common difficulties, and ways of overcoming them, include the following:

- Difficulty wringing out a flannel – use the taps to turn the cloth against, or use a small flannel and wring with one hand.
- Putting soap on a flannel – put the soap on a suctioned soap dish and wipe flannel over the soap.
- Difficulty reaching some areas of the body – use a long-handled sponge or brush.
- Getting in and out of the bath – use a bath board, seat with non-slip mat and grab bars.
- Fatigue – in the shower use a shower cradle or plastic chair and a long shower spray hose to make rinsing easier. Use a towelling robe to soak up water on the body and pat the body dry.
- Cleaning nails – use a suction nailbrush.
- Cleaning teeth or dentures – use a suction denture brush or electric toothbrush.
- Difficulty reaching round the back to put arm in sleeve – put on like a jumper. Also, as a general rule, put 'bad' arm in first when dressing and take out last when undressing, and use elasticated cuffs to provide give for fingers.

- Difficulty with fastenings because of poor motor control – replace with Velcro® or larger fastenings. Attach large loops to zippers. Fastening bras – change to front opening or fasten and put on like a jumper.
- Reaching difficulty – lower the rod in the wardrobe for ease of access. Use an 'easy reach' for picking up items that are hard to reach.
- Poor grip and range of motion – use long-handled, angled or broad-handled brushes and combs.
- Difficulty tying shoes – learn a one-handed method or use elasticated laces that are permanently tied, and use a long-handled shoe horn.

LEVELS OF INTERVENTION

A study by Booth *et al.* (2001) identifies four levels of intervention that can be used to rate the style and the nature of interventions used in assisting patients to wash and dress:

1. *Supervision.* Observing the patient and their activities with the purpose of ensuring the rehabilitative effects of each action or maintaining safety.

2. *Prompting/instructing.* Any non-physical communication between the helper and the patient that is intended to assist the patient in completing the activity attempted.

3. *Providing articles.* This includes providing washing and grooming equipment, preparation of clothing, and any other necessary equipment. The patient, using the equipment, carries out the actual activities.

4. *Facilitation.* Calculated use of the equipment or activity to facilitate the patient's movements, for example putting a limb through a natural movement sequence prior to the patient attempting the activity.

BATHING AND SHOWERING EQUIPMENT

Adjustable-height baths

Adjustable-height baths not only meet hygiene needs but also have an overall therapeutic effect if used well and if safe

Table 8.1 Potential deficits of different neurological conditions that may affect independence in washing and dressing.

	Sensory	Motor	Perceptual/cognitive
Brain injury/stroke	Loss of sensation of hot/cold Loss of sensation of touch pressure or pain Shoulder pain or central pain	Hemiplegia Poor balance and co-ordination Spasticity or contracture Flaccidity or weakness	Impaired attention, memory, planning and sequencing movements Body image/scheme deficit/apraxia Spatial relations deficit Depression
Multiple sclerosis	Hypersensitivity of temperature Exaggerated response to stimuli Neuropathic pain Visual disturbances	Weakness Spasticity Fatigue Problems with balance and posture	Memory loss Impaired reasoning and judgement Slower information processing Attention and concentration lapses Visuo-spatial perception may be impaired Depression
Parkinson's disease	Postural hypotension and dizziness Fainting	Tremor Slow, clumsy movements Difficulty initiating movement Arrests of ongoing movement Rigidity with increased muscle tone and stiffness Postural instability Fatigue	Depression Slowed thought processes Hallucination related to drug therapy Loss of memory and other cognitive functions
Dementia	Loss of sensory processing May be susceptible to being overstimulated	Reduced postural control Wandering and restlessness Loss of co-ordination and motor skill, manipulation and dexterity	Memory impairment Apraxia Agnosia Impaired planning, organisation, sequencing and topographical orientation Delusions, fearful, or aggressive
Epilepsy			Partial seizure activity may interfere with memory and concentration

techniques and procedures are followed. A good bathing system offers a wide choice of features and options to facilitate individualised care. The size and shape of the bath should be compatible with different types of lifting equipment (Dean 1998; Fitzgerald 1999; Collins 2001).

Shower trolleys

Shower trolleys are designed for showering patients in a lying position (see Figure 8.1). Patients can be transferred from a bed to a shower and back to bed without the need for further transfers. The mattress should be soft and wide to enhance patient comfort and allow for turning to wash the back. There should be safety latches to prevent accidental opening of the gates.

A shower trolley can be very useful in a room that has a showerhead and a plug to let the water drain away. Its use does

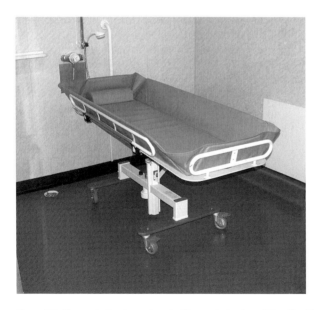

Figure 8.1 Shower trolley (reproduced with permission from Priory Healthcare).

not depend on a specially constructed bathroom, the main requirement being sufficient space to allow its entry and exit from the room.

The advantages of this type of equipment (Medical Devices Agency 1999; Thornley 2002) are:

- takes patients from bed to shower in one smooth operation;
- comfortable to lie on;
- easy access to the whole body;
- adjusts to comfortable working height;
- available in different sizes;
- works with a shower panel;
- very useful in non specialist areas;
- can be used with other patients.

Lift bath trolley

A lift bath trolley can be used with patients who are unable to sit up. It transports patients from the bed and lowers them into the bath in a comfortable position by bending in the middle. After bathing, the trolley can raise the patient from the bath and back to bed without any further transfers. It can have a moveable head pillow that allows transfers from either side of the bed. It does, however, need to be matched with a bath that allows clearance of the feet and raising equipment.

The advantages of this type of equipment are:

- only transfers from the bed and back again are needed;
- allows full immersion of the body;
- patients are in a sitting position and more likely to be able to participate.

Shower cradles

Shower cradles are tubular steel cradles with a supportive mesh sling and can be used to shower patients with some upper limb and trunk function, who have tracheostomies or who have very abnormal postures (see Figure 8.2).

The advantages of this type of equipment are that:

- it allows patients with poor sitting balance to be supported while showering and relearning independence.

- it can help release contractures and spasticity in the lower limbs while showering a patient.
- it allows access to all parts of the body using the stimulation of running water and allowing thorough rinsing.

Anwah (see case study in the section on How to Use this Book) seems to be very vulnerable and has little control, so whatever system is used in helping to maintain her hygiene, every opportunity for her to participate needs to be recognised. Participation confers a sense of control and choice: for example, choosing a shower where she can hold the showerhead and either independently or with direction shower herself. Routines can be established to reduce anxiety, and she can be given clear, concise explanations of what is going to happen, advising on every step to avoid alarming her and seeking agreement and confirmation from her that she is comfortable. Several options may be available. A shower cradle may be useful in that it will allow her to use her upper body function, be able to see more clearly what is going on around her and feel more in control of

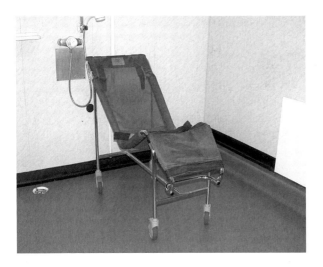

Figure 8.2 Shower cradle (reproduced with permission from Priory Healthcare).

what is happening. A shower cradle may make her feel safer as she is cocooned and has a sense of where her body is in space. If a shower cradle is not available, a shower trolley may be used, in that it allows the person to go from bed to shower in one easy movement, it has protective sides that may be reassuring to her. However, in this flat position she will be unable to use her upper body function, unable to help develop her sitting balance and will have the nurse looking down on her. A lift bath trolley is unsuitable because she cannot sit without support. A hoist with a bathing sling that holds her in a sitting position may be appropriate in this situation. If the ward does not have suitable equipment, several manufacturers offer a hiring option and it would be worth finding out about local policies and procedures with regard to hiring equipment.

Bath benches and seats, grab rails
Bath seats may be static or may raise and lower the patient into the bath and must be fitted or clamped securely to the bath. Non-skid mats should be outside the bathtub, avoiding the towel-type mat, which can be very unstable during transfers. Rubber safety treads should be suctioned to the bath floor, and safety grab rails should be fitted on the wall next to the bathtub or clamped to the edge of the bathtub. The rails may be straight or angled. This equipment can facilitate good independence but the patient's ability and co-ordination must be carefully assessed, as the transfers may be hazardous for them. Having a person seated while bathing or showering is safer for patients with poor balance or muscle weakness and is more energy efficient.

Other washing aids
- *Hand-held showers* – this showerhead attaches to a long hose which can be adapted for different types of taps.
- *Long-handled sponges* may come with a pocket to hold soap and angled for cleaning the back.
- *Wash mitts* made out of terry cloth have a Velcro® wrist closure and a loop that can be used to hang the mitt for drying. These can be used with liquid soap to eliminate the need to handle soap frequently.

- *Suction brushes* can be attached to the side of the bath or wash hand basin for cleaning fingernails.
- *Soap-on-a rope* can be worn around the neck or hung over a bath or shower fixture to keep it within easy reach.
- *Taps* may be fitted with levers to facilitate turning on and off. The cold tap should always be switched on first and hot water added gradually.

Louise (see case study in the section on How to Use this Book) has a sensory disturbance so the water temperature of the bath and the shower should be checked. She would probably need sensitive supervision, and could be offered some of the above washing aids to minimise fatigue. Fatigue may strongly influence her independence in this activity and be exacerbated by the side effects of her drug treatment and the intense humidity of the bathroom. She may need physical assistance to dry herself, and may wish to rest before she continues to dress.

Grooming aids and equipment
- *Nail care.* An emery board, nail clippers and nail files can be glued to a board to facilitate nail care.
- *Shaving.* An electric razor is safer than a blade razor for patients with incoordination. A strap around the razor can help prevent its being dropped. If it has a long flex, it can be used in places other than the bathroom. The shaver can be gripped by the knees to open the cover or remove the blade unit for cleaning. If a safety razor is used, a universal cuff and weighted wrist cuffs can give greater control for someone with poor coordination, weakness or tremors.
- *Hair care.* Hair drying can be easier and facilitate independence if the hair dryer is wall mounted or on an adjustable stand. There are many designs of curved, long-handled brushes and combs that help reach the back of the head, and some handles have interchangeable heads.
- *Oral hygiene.* An electric toothbrush may be more easily managed than an ordinary one. A standard toothbrush can be fitted with a universal cuff for someone with impaired grasp. Suction-cupped dentures can help to clean dentures, and denture pots can be lodged on non-slip matting. There are also

adaptive aids for squeezing toothpaste or hand cream from a tube using either a key turn or a lever handle technique, or some off-the-shelf dispensers require only palm pressure.
- *Deodorants.* There are several different types of adaptors for aerosol cans, most of which are interchangeable, or large roll-on deodorants could be used.

DRESSING

Although several assistive devices can help maintain independent dressing, neurological deficits need to be assessed and a dressing strategy developed that is both therapeutic and efficient. There is, however, a range of adaptive clothing that is widely used by people with neurological impairments.

- *Fastenings.* Front fasteners and stretch or loose-fitting fabric can help wheelchair users. For people with reduced sensation in the hands or lacking fine motor skills, Velcro fasteners are easier than buttons or zips, and elastic waistbands are easier than those that fasten. Where there are zips, loops on the tab or a curved hook can facilitate opening and closing. A button-hook with a large, weighted handle may be helpful. Men may find a clip-on tie easier, but tying the tie may be part of the therapeutic programme. Women may find front-fastening or slipover bras easier to use than ones that fasten at the back.
- *Fit.* Clothing one size larger than usual or stretch fitting will be easier to put on and large pockets are useful for carrying things in.
- *Footwear.* Elastic shoelaces, Velcro fastening or other adapted shoe closure or slip-on shoes eliminate the need to tie bows. Shoes may also offer support and stability as well as providing a safe, non-slip contact surface with the floor. Trainers are good for this purpose. Long-handled shoehorns, sock aids and wide-ankled, elasticised socks can all help reduce fatigue in lower body dressing.

ASSESSMENT OF WASHING AND DRESSING

For many neurological patients the involvement of an occupational therapist in developing a plan of care is the most effective way of establishing good habits and patterns. However, nurses are also important in dealing with this activity on a day-to-day basis. A thorough assessment of patients' sensory, motor, perceptual and cognitive ability is necessary as well as an appreciation of their psychosocial attitudes and cultural preferences. Even a seemingly simple activity such as brushing one's teeth involves a complex sequence of motor movements, using several large and small muscle groups in a co-ordinated series of flexions and extensions, as well as sensory experiences of the toothbrush and toothpaste in the mouth, all of which are co-ordinated and integrated by cognitive and perceptual integrity.

An assessment should take account of the following (Hecktor and Touhy 1997; Hoeffer *et al.* 1997; Collins 2001):

- Assess the level of help and type of equipment needed.
- Will the equipment need to be hired or purchased?
- Consider investing in a shower trolley, which is useful for a wide range of patients with mobility problems.
- Does the patient have flexion contractures that interfere with meeting the hygiene needs of any part of the body?
- How many people will be needed in bathing or showering this patient? Which type of sling needs to be used with the hoist?
- Suitable equipment can reduce the number of people needed in caring for people with poor mobility.
- What effects do the temperature, water or jet spray stimuli have on the patient's body? Unnecessary extremes of temperature and movement can trigger spasticity. A study by Widar *et al.* (2002) found that cold was the factor most increasing neuropathic pain following a stroke.
- Does the time of day affect the patient's ability to tolerate bath or shower, cradle or trolley?
- What are the effects on patients of the other sensory inputs (for example, smell of products, sounds within the bathroom, light reflection from the water, the feel of a toothbrush in their mouth)?

INTERVENTIONS

The aim is to meet hygiene needs and promote skin integrity using the bath or shower comfortably and safely. Interaction needs to encourage good movement patterns and to develop therapeutic sensory awareness.

- Negotiate with the patient in planning bathing and showering. Patient involvement increases autonomy and can reduce high tone due to fear or other negative moods. Bathing and showering opportunities help retrain sensory and perceptual experience in a relaxing activity.
- Use equipment that allows the patient to be transported comfortably and dried thoroughly without excessive temperature change. Extreme temperature change can cause painful spasticity.
- When possible, ensure that the body can be immersed. Full immersion stimulates blood flow and ensures that skin folds can be adequately cleaned.
- Fine temperature control prevents triggering of spasms.
- Foul-smelling areas of the body unable to be cleaned as a result of spasticity or contractures result from unacceptable care practice.
- Contact physiotherapy and medical staff or a specialist if spasticity or contracture makes access to any part of the body difficult.
- Use equipment that allows the patient to be transported comfortably and dried thoroughly.

PSYCHOSOCIAL ASPECTS

Neurological deficits are nearly always accompanied by a change in body image, and this can be exacerbated by the effect the impairments may have on the range and choice of clothes that people can wear and are suitable. People may need to change their clothes more frequently, may spill food and drink on their clothing and may no longer be able to wear the style of clothes to which they have become accustomed. Also, with some loss of independence they may feel they have lost some autonomy in choosing what to wear and ensuring favourite items are laundered as and when they want them. For example, jogging suits and trainers are often recommended during physiotherapy to allow freedom of movement and good non-slip contact with the floor. In addition, if there is cognitive impairment, people may have lost awareness of the social impact of grooming and appropriate clothing.

Nurses can assist patients to maintain as much dignity as possible by encouraging independence using adapted clothing, giving them the opportunity to make choices, complimenting their appearance, and giving tactful feedback and sensitive intervention when patients have difficulty presenting themselves as they would wish.

SUMMARY
❏ Motor problems, sensory problems and perceptual problems such as agnosia, apraxia and deficits in recognising spatial relationships, and cognitive problems such as maintaining attention, self-monitoring and self-evaluation can affect independence in washing, dressing and grooming and can affect a person's sense of dignity, individuality, autonomy and social belonging.
❏ Several levels of intervention can be used following assessment of a person's need. These include supervision, prompting/instructing, providing article and adapted equipment and clothing, and facilitation.
❏ The bathing and showering equipment used has a strong influence on patient safety, level of independence and fatigue. Equipment includes adjustable-height baths, shower trolleys, shower cradles, lift bath trolleys, bath benches, seats and grab rails, and modified nailbrushes, hand mitts or taps. Many neurological patients have strong sensitivity to the rapid changes of temperature in bathing and showering.
❏ Patients may feel embarrassed and need encouragement to develop positive attitudes to accepting the need for modification of their usual and preferred style of clothing, and advice on suitable fastenings, fit and stretchiness of fabric.

REFERENCES
Booth, J., Davidson, I., Winstanley, J. and Waters, K. (2001) Observing washing and dressing of stroke patients: nursing interventions compared with occupational therpaists. What is the difference? *Journal of Advanced Nursing* **33** (1), 98–105.

Collins, F. (2001) Choosing bathing, showering and toileting equipment. *Nursing and Residential Care* **3** (10), 488–9.

Dean, R. (1998) Considerations for bathroom equipment and adaptations. *British Journal of Therapy and Rehabilitation* **5** (1), 13–16.

Edmans, J., Champion, A., Hill, L. *et al.* (2001) *Occupational Therapy and Stroke.* Whurr, London.

Fitzgerald, J. (1999) The new Neptune bathlift from Mountway. *Nursing and Residential Care* **1** (2), 116–18.

Hecktor, L. M. and Touhy, T. A. (1997) The history of the bath: from art to task? Reflections for the future. *Journal of Gerontological Nursing* **23** (5), 7–15.

Hoeffer, B., Rader, J., McKenzie, D., Lavelle, M. and Stewart, B. (1997) Reducing aggressive behaviour during bathing cognitively impaired nursing home residents. *Journal of Gerontological Nursing* **23** (5), 16–23.

Medical Devices Agency (1999) *Bathing and Showering Equipment for People with Severe Disabilities,* (EL3) MDA. Department of Health, London.

Thornley, H. (2002) Product focus: the new Neptune bathlift from Mountway. *British Journal of Therapy and Rehabilitation* **9** (10), 401–3.

Widar, M., Samuelsson, L., Karlsson-Tivenius, S. and Ahlstrom, G. (2002) Long-term pain conditions after stroke. *Journal of Rehabilitaiton Medicine* **34** (4), 165–70.

Controlling Body Temperature

9

INTRODUCTION

Although it is unlikely in a general setting that neurological patients will suffer from critically unstable temperature control caused by neurological damage, the impairments they do have can make them more vulnerable to chest and urinary infection and hypersensitive to temperature change. The presence of a fever in patients with a neurological impairment can worsen their neurological symptoms, cause confusion, interfere with a valid neurological assessment, cause discomfort and interfere with lifestyle. Lack of awareness of hypersensitivity to temperature change on the part of the nurse can cause painful and disabling cramps and spasticity in the patient, and in the case of hyposensitivity can lead to skin damage and scalding. Nursing interventions in this activity need to be based on a good assessment of the underlying problems, its triggers and effects, and may develop over time as nurses become more familiar with the patient, enabling them to help alleviate the problem and increase patient comfort.

The aim of this chapter is to draw attention to the mechanisms of temperature control in the body, how these can be affected by neurological impairment and the interventions nurses can use to help minimise the effect of impaired body temperature control.

LEARNING OUTCOMES

❑ Understand the role of the hypothalamus in regulating body temperature centrally.

❑ Discuss the neurological impairments that can lead to altered perception of body temperature, altered homeostasis or increased risk of infection.

❏ Outline effective care planning to minimise the effects of neurological damage on temperature balance and prevent infection from developing.
❏ Outline effective care planning to minimise the effect of pyrexia on neurological function.

TEMPERATURE CONTROL MECHANISMS

Body temperature, like other physical measures, has a normal range into which most people will fall. It tends to be higher in younger people, after physical exercise or a large meal, in the evening and at different stages of the menstrual cycle (Axford and O'Callaghan 2004). Body heat is detected by temperature-sensitive cells in the hypothalamus, which then stimulate the autonomic system to initiate heat-losing mechanisms such as flushing, sweating and thirst, or heat-gaining mechanisms such as shivering and narrowing of the blood vessels near the surface of the skin to conserve heat for vital body organs. During a fever, the temperature setting of the hypothalamus is altered by chemical messengers from the immune system and allows the set point to increase to as far as approximately 40.5°C (Kunihiro and Foster 1998). This increase allows the metabolic rate to rise to the level required to quickly increase defensive white cells. This explains why, as the temperature is rising, the body uses a heat-producing mechanism such as shivering in order to produce pyrexia.

The autonomic nerves regulate peripheral body temperature. These act on the skin and small blood vessels, sweat glands and other skin receptors to retain or lose heat peripherally when the environmental temperature is high or exercise has produced more body heat (Marieb 1999). This peripheral response is not reflected by a change in the temperature of the blood or organs, known as the core temperature. There should be no more than 3°C difference between the core temperature and the peripheral temperature.

Hyperpyrexia

Temperatures that reach beyond 41°C are hyperpyrexic; they may damage brain cell function and result in associated fits or rigors (Hickey 1997; Jamieson *et al.* 2002). Pyrexia up to 40°C inhibits bacterial and viral growth (Ganong 1995), amplifies the immune response and promotes tissue repair (Rowsey 1997; Woodrow 2000).

Hyperpyrexia is the result of the loss of hypothalamic control because one of the following has occurred:

• The mechanisms for heat loss are overwhelmed, as in heatstroke.
• Activity inside the body is producing heat too fast, as in status epilepticus or thyrotoxic crisis, or in systemic infections such as meningitis or septicaemia. This is a very dangerous development and the temperature can rise out of control very rapidly.
• The function of the hypothalamus itself has been damaged by an intracranial haemorrhage (stroke), tumour or traumatic injury. This is a serious development in people with a brain injury since it increases the metabolic rate and therefore the oxygen demand on the brain. This can lead to ischaemia in the brain, raising the intracranial pressure and causing further damage.

Hypothermia
Hypothermia is defined as a core temperature of less than 35°C and occurs when the body loses too much heat or cannot maintain its normothermic state (Jevon and Ewens 2002).

Neurological patients may be at risk of developing hypothermia as a result of:

• spinal shock when autonomic innervation is lost, although this is usually after trauma;
• metabolic or toxic coma of any origin, including alcohol;
• drug overdose, particularly from barbiturates, benzodiazepines;
• impaired perception of body temperature as in dementia or other perceptual disorders such as body scheme or neglect of one side of the body as in hemiplegia;
• exposure to a cold environment, poor accommodation, poor mobility and malnourishment.

Monitoring patients with hypo- and hyperthermia
Monitoring should include regular assessment of vital signs, arterial blood gas analysis to make sure acidosis is not developing, ECG monitoring to detect arrhythmias, urine output and fluid balance recording, blood sugar estimations and neurological observations (Jevon and Ewens 2002). Cooling measures should be cautious and both core and skin temperature measured to avoid overshoot hypothermia and rebound hyperthermia (Aun 1997). These observations should also be made if a patient is hypothermic and being warmed.

Autonomic disturbances in temperature control mechanisms

Sometimes disturbances of the autonomic system, as in a neuropathy such as Guillain-Barré, may manifest as signs of disturbed body temperature control. These may include partial or complete loss of sweating, and heat intolerance, which may involve the person feeling hot, flushed, dizzy and weak without sweating (Harati 1998). Other discomforts may include excessive sweating, or sweating when eating food or at night. Disturbance of the normal function of the autonomic nervous system is called *dysautomnia*.

Hypersensitivity
Damage to the myelin sheath, as in multiple sclerosis, may cause hypersensitivity to the temperature changes involved in moving from the bedroom to the bathroom into the bath water and then to the cooling effects of the water on skin as the patient emerges from the bath. Also, the heat and water vapour in the bathroom may increase fatigue, further exacerbate hypersensitivity and increase sensitivity to pain.

Hyposensitivity
Hyposensitivity may occur in patients with traumatic or acquired brain injury, with neuropathies that cause numbness or with spinal cord injury. Such patients may be at risk of being scalded or burnt because of lost sensation.

Louise (see case study in the section on How to Use this Book) may be particularly affected by these autonomic disturbances, showing hypersensitivity to water temperature or to shower pressure, or she may have insensitivity to heat and be in danger of scalding herself. Anwah (see case study) may have some autonomic disturbance of body temperature control as a result of her brain damage and may need protection from the rapid changes of temperature during bathing and showering.

OTHER POTENTIAL SOURCES OF DISTURBED TEMPERATURE

- Swallowing problems and immobility may lead to chest infections because of silent aspiration. Irene (see case study in the section on How to Use this Book) may be particularly prone to this as she already has breathing problems and there is some concern about her swallowing efficiency. Fred (see case study) may also be vulnerable because of his considerably reduced mobility and potential for poor saliva control and poor mastication.
- Neurogenic bladder may cause urinary infection because of high residual volumes of urine, to which Louise is particularly vulnerable.
- Central and peripheral lines tracheal and gastrostomy tubes may become a focus of infection.
- Urinary catheters may lead to recurrent infections.
- Steroid therapy. The anti-inflammatory agents used to suppress inflammation in some neurological conditions often mask the classical signs of infection, so careful observation is needed to monitor for other signs of a developing infection. For example, if Louise is being treated with steroids for relapse of her multiple sclerosis, the treatment may mask a urinary tract infection caused by retention and stasis or introduced with intermittent self-catheterisation.
- Autonomic dysreflexia, which may include sweating or flushing without infection, which is discussed in Chapter 2.

MEASURING BODY TEMPERATURE

Since the introduction of the Control of Substances Hazardous to Health (COSHH) regulations, glass mercury thermometers are no longer used in the UK, having been replaced by electronic or chemical dot thermometry (Walker 2004). For neurological patients, the oral cavity is very often an inappropriate location for recording the core temperature, and the tympanic membrane in the ear is a suitable alternative.

Electronic probes with a single-use disposable sleeve reduces the risk of cross-infection between patients and do not carry the risk of glass thermometers (Edwards 1997). They may be used in the axilla, oral cavity or rectum.

Chemical dot thermometers are also single-use and consist of a thin plastic strip with dots of thermosensitive chemicals that change colour to show the correct temperature.

Tympanic thermometers use infrared radiation, using a probe and a disposable cover, to measure the temperature of blood flowing through the tympanic membrane of the ear. It is considered accurate, as it is close to the hypothalamus and shares its blood supply.

Research findings, however, are inconclusive (Sganga *et al.* 2000) about the most accurate instrument to use. Reliability can be achieved by making sure that the same instrument is used on the same patient each time the temperature is taken. The choice of equipment and route is a clinical one and the principles for temperature recording can normally be adapted for any type of thermometer (Fulbrook 1993).

NURSING ASSESSMENT

Points to consider when assessing and planning care might include the following:

- Are there any particular neurological impairments that might cause difficulty in homeostasis?
- Are there any impairments or deficits that might interfere with peripheral sensation of hot and cold?
- Does the person have hypersensitivity to a change in room temperature or environmental temperature?
- Does the person have perceptual or cognitive impairments that might affect perception or behavioural response to a change in temperature?

- Is the person able to detect or control temperature changes in the environment?
- Can the person make appropriate choices and take appropriate actions?

NURSING INTERVENTIONS

The evidence base for nursing interventions for managing fever is not strong (While 2000), and is not specific to the circumstances of neurological patients. The general principles of pyrexia management due to infection is to allow the body temperature to reach the new level set by the hypothalamus. This may include using blankets when the patient is shivering and facilitating the loss of body heat when the body tries to lose heat naturally. Other measures include the following:

- Screening for the sites of infection, including taking specimens and wound swabs.
- Administering acetaminophin (650 mg every 4–6 hours as needed).
- Giving tepid water baths and tepid sponging. In the chill phase of systemic fever, cooling measures such as tepid sponging are not appropriate as cooling the shell of the body will encourage further generation of heat (Casey 2000). It is preferable to use antipyretic medications such as paracetamol. Tepid sponging achieves heat loss by evaporation of heat from the moist skin surface. For evaporation to occur, the body must be hotter than the temperature of the surrounding environment (Watson 1998). Tepid sponging can be used if it helps the patient to feel more comfortable and there are no neurological contraindications.
- Avoiding shivering which may further derange homeostasis. Electric fans may be used to carry body heat away from the surface of the body – this is the same effect as wind chill (Watson 1998). Fans, however, should not be directed on to the patient's skin as this may induce shivering because of vasoconstriction, a heat-producing mechanism. In addition, fans may be reservoirs of infection.
- Removal of excess bedcovers. In the flush and diaphoresis phases, nursing interventions facilitate loss of body heat.

- Ensuring that environmental temperatures are ambient and stable at around 20°C.
- Ensuring clear fluid intake of around 2 litres per day.

The difficulties in implementing these strategies with neurological patients centre on gaining co-operation, balancing heat loss tactics with hypersensitive responses and ensuring adequate oral fluid intake if enteral tube feeding has not been initiated. For example, if Fred develops a chest or urinary infection, his mental clarity and his co-operation will be further clouded. Extra measures to ensure a good fluid intake may need to be initiated because of his increased off periods and he may need any prescribed antibiotics as an elixir to help ensure that he swallows it all and gets the full benefit of the course.

INTERVENTIONS TO MANAGE HYPOTHERMIA
Depending on the cause, specific treatments may include:

- warming blankets;
- raising the temperature of the room;
- monitoring patients at risk because of altered perception of body and environmental temperature.

Wandering patients can be a particular problem as they may be wearing nightclothes suitable for sleeping in a bed but not for wandering around in. If wandering is a problem, the main aim is to cover the body surface area to minimise heat loss and to gain advantage from the extra heat generated by the movements.

PREVENTING HYPERSENSITIVE RESPONSES TO CHANGES IN TEMPERATURE
Sudden changes in temperature can stimulate spasticity in neurological patients, leading to spasms, pain, difficulty in carrying out activities, and fatigue. This can be a particular problem during washing and dressing, and every effort needs to be made to avoid provoking this. For example, nurses could ensure that Anwah is covered with a blanket until the very last moment before she has a shower and that she is covered by warmed towels when she emerges. If she is going outside she will

need adequate clothing or blankets and she may need a heat exchanger over her tracheostomy tube to counter the coolness of the air outside.

SUMMARY

❏ The hypothalamus regulates body temperature centrally, allowing the core temperature to reset itself in the presence of infection to support the metabolic rate needed for the immune system to produce more cells.

❏ Acquired or traumatic brain damage, brain tumour or lesion affecting the hypothalamus can disrupt homeostatic mechanisms.

❏ Other neurological impairments such as dementia can lead to altered perception of body temperature and dysphagia; catheterisation can increase the risk of infection; and demyelination or inflammation of neurones can make people hypersensitive to external and internal changes in temperature.

❏ Sudden changes in environmental temperature should be minimised.

❏ When using body cooling or warming measures, take into account the person's neurological deficits and adapt measures if necessary.

❏ Screen potential sources of infection, taking swabs and specimens if indicated.

REFERENCES

Aun, C. (1997) Thermal disorders. In Oh, T. (ed.), *Intensive Care Manual*, 4th edn. Butterworth-Heinemann, Oxford.

Axford, J. and O'Callaghan, C. A. (2004) *Medicine*, 2nd edn. Blackwell, Oxford.

Casey, G. (2000) Fever management in children. *Paediatric Nursing* **12** (3), 38–43.

Edwards, S. (1997) Measuring temperature. *Professional Nurse* **13** (2), 253–8.

Fulbrook, P. (1993) Core temperature measurement: a comparison of rectal, axillary and pulmonary artery blood temperature. *Intensive and Critical Care Nursing* **9** (4), 43–4.

Ganong, W. (1995) *Review of Medical Physiology*, 17th edn. Prentice Hall, London.

Harati, Y. (1998) In: Rolak, L. A. (ed.) *Neurology Secrets*, 2nd edn. Hanley & Belfus, Philadelphia, chapter 4.

Hickey, J. (1997) *The Clinical Practice of Neurological and Neurosurgical Nursing*, 4th edn. Lippincott, Philadelphia.

Jamieson, E. M., McNall, J. M. and Whyte, L. A. (2002) *Clinical Nursing Practices*. Churchill Livingstone, Edinburgh.

Jevon, P. and Ewens, B. (2002) *Monitoring the Critically Ill Patient*. Blackwell Science, Oxford.

Kunihiro, A. and Foster, J. (1998) Heat exhaustion and heat stroke, available at http://www.emedicicne.com/EMERG/tropic236htm.HUman

Marieb, E. (1999) *Human Anatomy and Physiology*, 4th edn. Benjamin Cummings, California.

Rowsey, P. (1997) Pathophysiology of fever. Part 2: Relooking at cooling interventions. *Dimensions of Critical Care Nursing* **15** (5), 251–6.

Sganga, A., Wallace, R., Kiehl, E., Irving, T. and Witter, L. (2000) A comparison of four methods of normal newborn temperature measurement. *American Journal of Maternal/Child Nursing* **25** (2), 76–9.

Walker, S. (2004) Controlling body temperature. In: Holland, K., Jenkins, J., Solomon, J. and Whittam, S. (eds), *Applying the Roper, Logan and Tierney Model in Practice*. Churchill Livingstone, Edinburgh, chapter 9.

Watson, R. (1998) Controlling body temperature in adults. *Emergency Nurse* **6** (1), 31–9.

While, A. (2000) Putting fever in perspective. *British Journal of Community Nursing* **5** (10), 517.

Woodrow, P. (2000) *Intensive Care Nursing: A Framework for Practice*. Routledge, London.

Mobilising | **10**

INTRODUCTION

Impaired ability to move normally is one of the most common and profoundly distressing effects of neurological disease. Impairments may affect a person's ability to move freely, to use the face and body to express feelings and emotions and to be independent in carrying out activities of living basic to life. This can have a negative impact on the person's quality of life, interaction with others, and idea of self. For example, slowness of movement is often misinterpreted and incorrectly assumed to demonstrate impaired intelligence. This may be the case, but often it is not. In addition, others can interpret uncontrolled or apparently purposeless movement as corresponding with disturbed and bizarre thought processes, labelling the person as odd. Chapter 4 discusses further aspects of motor ability that can cause problems in interpersonal communication. In addition, paralysis and immobility increase dependence on others, which can often evoke patronising and impatient attitudes from other people. A holistic approach to care planning, working closely with physiotherapists and occupational therapists, can minimise disability and facilitate therapeutic interaction in practical daily life.

This chapter focuses on understanding the physical basis of normal movement, the effect that impairment has on a person's ability to carry out their life independently, and the strategies that nurses can use to reduce the effect of the impairment on the person's physical well-being, autonomy and social function.

LEARNING OUTCOMES

❑ Outline some basic concepts in discussing normal movement.
❑ Understand the meaning of the terms postural tone, key points of control, base of support.

❏ Describe how spasticity can be managed.
❏ Understand general principles in managing hemiplegia following acquired brain injury.
❏ Describe a range of equipment such as hoists, wheelchairs, tilt-in-space chairs, profiling beds, cushions and mattresses, and appreciate how clinical reasoning informs choice of selection.

NORMAL MOVEMENT

Normal movements are made up of patterns of muscle contraction and relaxation that help the body to make the movement and remain stable with a well-distributed muscle tone.

To move normally, a person needs to receive, integrate and respond appropriately to stimuli that come from a range of environmental, psychological, physiological, social and emotional sources. Although we all have individual style in moving, all movements derive from efficient patterns that we develop in infancy and as we add new motor skills to our repertoire. The patterns become automatic, such as walking or riding a bicycle, for example, once a pattern is well rehearsed.

In neurological disease, this automatic background is disrupted because of damage to the nerves supplying a muscle or group of muscles. Someone may still be able sit, stand or walk but with abnormal patterns of muscle activity (Hannah 1995; Johnstone 1995; Edwards 2002). Even when lying down the neurological damage can cause uneven and abnormal patterns of muscle activity. The abnormal posture can complicate and delay recovery. The patient should be positioned properly and rehearse good movement in every activity to correct abnormal patterns (see Table 10.1).

Postural tone

In addition to automatic patterns, smooth movements need the right *muscle tone.* Muscle tone is the readiness of the body's muscles to sustain a posture or carry out a movement. *Contracted muscle* has high tone, *relaxed muscle* has low tone, and both are affected by the condition of the nervous system, the condition of the muscles and the *base of support* for body weight. The base of support is the area of the body in contact with the

Table 10.1 Common deformities which can be corrected if caught early.

Abnormality	Cause	Prevention
Windsweeping	If a patient lies on their back for long periods with their knees flexed there is a strong tendency for the knees to fall to the side (either left or right). If the legs are not supported, this creates a position of abduction, external rotation at one hip and adduction internal rotation at the other	Use of the T-roll when supine (that is, lying on the back) in a neutral position – adds stability to the patient's position in bed
Flexion at the trunk and neck	This can develop over time if a patient who does not have the postural ability to maintain an upright posture against gravity is seated in an upright wheelchair chair. Over time, the position causes the head to drop and the upper trunk and neck to flex. This results in a poor position for communication, interaction with the environment, feeding etc.	An important method of correcting this is the use of the tilt-in-space wheelchair chair. The chair gives the patient a biomechanical advantage to counteract gravity and makes it easier to keep the head in an upright position as well as creating a more stable body posture
Extension and side flexion of the trunk	Following acquired brain injury some patients develop very high muscle tone in the extensor muscles causing a 'straightening' of the knees, hips, trunk and neck. This is often accompanied by side flexion of the trunk and neck	One method of preventing this from developing into fixed contracture is use of a supportive sleep system. This consists of blocks positioned in the bed to support the patient in a symmetrical position (see Figure 10.3 in the section on equipment, below) counteracting the pull of the muscle tone. In addition, it is important to sit the client out in an appropriate seating system

supporting surface. Usually a person is more stable when lying down than when sitting or standing since the base of support is more extensive. However, even when a person is lying down there are spinal reflexes that can generate abnormal postures. When a person is sitting or standing, normal postural tone needs to be high enough to maintain an upright posture against gravity and yet adaptable enough to maintain balance.

Muscle innervation

The nerves that supply muscles either generate a higher tone and contraction or inhibit tone, allowing the muscle to relax. They do this through the release of neurotransmitters that affect muscle activity, as shown in Chapter 1. Normal patterns of muscle innervation produce effective groups of contracted and relaxed muscles that facilitate joint movement. Damage to the brain, however, can derange the balance, and muscle tone can remain high because the inhibitory influence from the brain is lost, causing reduced range of motion. Abnormal posture that develops from the loss of inhibition can be minimised by breaking up the pattern. These positions are known as *inhibitory positions* (Johnstone 1991, 1995; Lynch and Grisogono 1991).

Spasms and cramps occur when neurones stimulate excessive muscle contraction, the strength of which prevents oxygen reaching the muscle tissue, causing spasm and cramping pains.

Balance, trunk control and sitting balance

Most of our daily movements involve balanced muscle activity of the trunk muscles, but neurological impairments, such as stroke, traumatic brain injury or motor neurone disease, can make sitting in a balanced position very effortful. To overcome this, patients use *compensatory movement strategies*, recruiting muscles that would not normally be involved in the pattern.

Proprioception and key points

Sensory information from touch, pressure, vision and *proprioception* also affect balancing reactions. People with neurological damage can be assisted to overcome abnormal patterns by facilitating the key points of control. Key point control facilitates normal movement by unlocking a movement pattern in the spine or lower brain (Rutishauser 1994; Kirker *et al.* 2000; Pollock *et al.* 2000; Edwards 2002).

SPASTICITY AND ITS MANAGEMENT

Spasticity is the loss of balanced muscle control and tone, giving some muscle groups excessively high tone. It is a common problem in most neurological diseases, and a particular problem after brain injury and in severe multiple sclerosis. Specialists in spasticity management have detailed knowledge of different kinds of spasticity. In most clinical practice settings, however, spasticity describes a state of high muscle tone that prevents normal movements or that interferes with activities of living and nursing care.

Normally, stretch receptors ensure that muscles do not shorten or stretch too much. In neurological disease or impairment, the effect of the upper motor neurones regulating the reflex and fine tuning muscle stimulation may be limited or lost (Johnstone 1995). As result, there is unchecked stimulation from the spinal cord to the muscle. There is an increase in muscle tone, with an exaggerated stretch reflex or unopposed overactivity of the flexor muscles. Limbs thus become rigid in an extensor or flexor pattern and resist attempts to alter the pattern.

Chronic spasticity can lead to the following changes in the muscles involved and in neighbouring muscles:

- the muscles waste and may fibrose;
- the tendons that connect the muscles to the joint shorten;
- the joint capsule may shrink;
- permanent contracture may develop (Edwards 2002).

In addition, bone can be laid down in the soft tissue outside the joint. This condition is called *heterotopic ossification*. It fixes a joint in an abnormal position, causing serious nursing and therapy problems.

Spasms may occur when moving, washing or dressing patients who have spasticity, and the severity and distribution of spasticity can vary enormously in different positions.

Severe spasticity and contractures often develop in the early stages of brain injury because of poor care (Carr and Shepherd 1998; Sullivan 2000; Harding 2001; Porter 2001), such as:

- poor positioning;
- failure to break spastic patterns;
- ineffective pain management;
- pressure sores;
- poor bowel and bladder management;

They can also develop as a result of fatigue, stress, irritation from clothing, catheter bags, or some medications and pain. Even patients with a very low cognitive level demonstrate primitive pain response such as hyperventilating, sweating, increased and severe spasms.

ANTISPASTICITY MEDICATION

The most popular oral medications include baclofen (Kamensek 1999a,b), tizanidine and Valium (diazepam). All decrease muscle tone, but they can also have undesirable effects such as drowsiness, weakness and floppiness. Dantrolene sodium is less likely to cause these effects but it can be toxic to the liver. These side effects may interfere with progress, and local treatment such as botulinum toxin can be used instead. It is effective and has few side effects beyond slight local muscle weakness (Kimiur 1997; Dressler 2000; Barnes and Johnson 2001; Elovic and Zafonte 2001; Turner-Stokes and Ward 2002; Taricco *et al.* 2003).

A further disadvantage of oral antispasticity medication is that it can lower the seizure threshold in brain-injured patients and sudden cessation can result in withdrawal seizures (Gracies *et al.* 1997). For this reason, patients should be weaned off oral antispasticity agents gradually. Nurses also have a responsibility in monitoring the effects of antispasticity treatment, noting its effectiveness or side effects throughout the activities of living. A checklist should include the following questions:

- Is the overall tone lowered too much?
- Have the person's attention and concentration been affected?
- Does the dose need to be adjusted (responses to the medication are highly individual)?
- What nursing observations need to be made?
- How are they to be recorded and reported?

JOYCE'S CASE

Joyce (see case study in the section on How to Use this Book) clearly needs review of her spasticity management by specialist medical and physiotherapy staff.

Nursing interventions

Nursing staff have a responsibility to report to the specialist staff the extent to which the uncontrolled spasticity is affecting Joyce's progress. Nurses would be able to evaluate the effects of oral baclofen during normal bedside care activities, and whether an increased dose gave better muscle stretching, better passive movement response, and reduced pain spasm and tightness, or whether the dose produced undesirable side effects such as weakness, drowsiness, floppiness, dizziness or even confusion. Nurses can also ensure that spasticity is minimised by making sure that Joyce is lying and sitting in inhibitory positions that can help decrease the stimulus to the affected muscle. In addition, unpleasant stimulation such as pain, constipation, catheter bags, stress, fatigue, fear, temperature extremes or sudden movements can all be minimised to help prevent a spastic trigger.

Botulinum toxin

For Joyce, botulinum toxin injections may be the best option. It is a powerful neurotoxin that is diluted in saline and injected directly into the spastic muscle. There it blocks the release of substance from the damaged nerves that would tend to increase muscle tone. Because this substance is now blocked, relaxation of the muscle begins to be seen over subsequent days. The drug can do this without affecting the more distant muscles. The effect lasts for two to three months. After that time the effect wears off because of the axonal sprouting of the peripheral nerve and re-innervation of the muscle. The dose can be adjusted to the degree of weakness needed to overcome the spasticity. It is effective in both large and small muscles and many patients experience less pain after injection. The side effects are minimal, the main one being that it may not work. Others are muscle weakness due to over-relaxation and the possibility of some slight leakage of botulinum toxin into the surrounding tissue. For Joyce, however, it is an ideal option. It would give her the length of time needed to continue her rehabilitation and progress in all her activities.

SURGICAL INTERVENTIONS

Surgical interventions may be made when all else fails. Neurosurgeons operate on the sensory nerve roots in the spinal column. This prevents sensory nerves from sending excitatory messages to the motor nerve and thus generating high muscle tone. Orthopaedic surgeons can lengthen, release or transfer contracted or spastic muscle, or can operate on a joint fixed by heterotopic ossification (Perry 1999).

COMMON PROBLEMS IN HEMIPLEGIA

Following a stroke or traumatic brain injury, one side of the body may be impaired by weakness, flaccidity and spasticity. The problems that ensue include:

- problems with body symmetry in the trunk, making sitting balance difficult, with shift of weight to either the affected side or the unaffected side;
- head may be flexed to the affected side;
- loss of range of motion in some major joints;
- change in muscle tone depending on body position;
- loss of skilled motor movement pattern on the affected side;
- disordered movement pattern;
- loss of automatic reflexes, balancing mechanism, sense of position;
- loss of motor planning and the ability to interpret the position of body parts in relation to space and in relation to each other;
- perceptual impairments that lead to neglect of body parts, impaired judgement of spatial relations, depth and distance.

ELLA'S CASE

Ella (see case study in the section on How to Use this Book) has a dense right hemiplegia and this may present as flaccid in the early stages, but may be followed by spasticity as time goes on. She will need assistance to change position and a profiling bed will help with this. When she is lying on her affected side her shoulder should be brought forward, with her arm at a right angle to her body, the affected hip extended and the knee flexed, supported in this position if necessary with pillows. This inhibitory position will normalise muscle tone, improve symmetry and help prevent contracture. She has altered sensation on her right side and she is at high risk of pressure damage on this side of her body. Ella can only sit out if the physiotherapist agrees that her sitting balance is good enough, and the nurse needs to liaise closely with the physiotherapist. If the physiotherapist agrees that Ella can sit out, this should only be for short periods, as rest and correct positioning are very important post-stroke. The back and the seat of the chair should support Ella's body in a 90 degree angle, with both hips flexed and feet flat on the floor or footrest.

ROLE OF THE PHYSIOTHERAPIST
In assessing altered motor ability, physiotherapy aims to reduce excessive muscle tone and restore as normal patterns of movement as possible or to teach safe compensatory strategies. This involves:

- assessing the patterns of movement;
- finding inhibitory positions, postures and movements;
- ensuring that the range of movement and muscle tone are maintained by stretching exercises which nurses can supervise;
- if necessary, using splints to correct excessively high tone.

PHYSIOTHERAPY APPROACHES TO MANAGING DISTURBED NORMAL MOVEMENT
In mobilising, physiotherapists provide guidance on the following aspects of treatment and care:

- Correct positioning and posture, in lying and sitting to manage tone and feedback.
- Effective handling techniques that make use of the key points of control to unlock normal movement patterns and to return the centre of gravity to the midline when balance is disturbed.

- Maintaining the range of movements in joints, maintaining muscle length and preventing contracture through range-of-movement exercises, passive stretches and splinting. Casts may be replaced as the limb progressively repositions, or a soft splint may be made from a material such as Lycra® which gives both support and limited movement to the joint.
- Advising on any equipment needed, and the level and type of assistance to give when patients are transferring or walking.
- Maximising function and preventing secondary complications in patients with progressive and chronic conditions by teaching patients exercise programmes so that they can take part in maintaining their own range of movement and muscle power (Watkins 1999; Kilbride and McDonnell 2000; Ada and Dwyer 2001; Grissom and Blanton 2001; Stockmann 2001; Harvey *et al.* 2002; Harvey and Herbert 2002).

ROLE OF THE OCCUPATIONAL THERAPIST

Occupational therapists help patients to redevelop living skills using the physical readiness that the physiotherapist helps to create and by modifying the person's movements in carrying out their activities (Wallen 1995). They carry out a detailed analysis of the movement patterns for daily activities upon which to base interventions using aids and equipment, energy conservation, safety and activity simplification techniques. For example, an activity analysis by an occupational therapist can indicate changes such as where items are kept on a shelf, in a drawer or locker to avoid having to stand on toes, extend trunk and stretch that may challenge balance mechanisms. They may recommend strategies to reduce fatigue and conserve energy, such as type of seating, positioning devices and support systems required to carry out an activity comfortably and safely.

Occupational therapists also assess a patient's cognitive and perceptual abilities and impairments, helping them to develop strategies to overcome impairments of attention, memory or concentration which may be impeding their physical recovery (Atwood 1999; Reed 2001).

USING WORKING SPACE AND EQUIPMENT EFFECTIVELY

Planning mobility care using mechanical aids and effective techniques in the short and long term has considerable benefits for patients, nursing staff and carers (Hannah 1995; Berg 1998; Hartshorn 2001). These benefits include:

- patients who are fresher, more active with a maintained quality of life and are psychologically motivated;
- greater work safety and work satisfaction for staff with reduced strain;
- promotion of optimum mobility for patients maintaining the capacity of the heart, lungs and blood circulation.
- reducing the risk of pneumonia, thrombosis, incontinence, urinary tract infection, pressure sores and dizziness.

TYPES OF EQUIPMENT

Beds and mattresses

A four-section profiling adjustable bed provides pressure relief by its variable posture mechanism.

- By changing the profile of the bed, the patient's position and weight distribution will change, which will help to break up spastic patterns.
- The knee-break helps to reduce shearing forces and prevents users from slipping down the bed.
- The patient can easily assume a sitting position in bed by the variable height and angle of the adjustable backrest.

Profiling beds can be used in conjunction with a pressure-reducing foam mattress or viscoelastic mattress that minimises the pressure by conforming to the shape of the body and reducing the effects of shear forces and friction. An air- or fluid-filled bed is unstable because of the ever-changing base of support. This can cause unwanted activity in muscle groups and may cause feelings of insecurity. As long as frequent positional changes are made, a conforming mattress contours to the body well and confers a feeling of security (Gray *et al.* 1997; Hampton 1998; Mitchell *et al.* 1998; O'Connor 2000; Rithalia and Kenney 2000; Russell 2001; Cullum *et al.* 2002).

The use of airflow mattresses in neurological patients for preventing pressure sores should be discussed with a physiotherapist, balancing the gains in pressure relief against the potentially adverse effects on muscle tone and posture of the alternating base of support.

T-Rolls

T-rolls are inexpensive foam rolls shaped as a T which, when inserted beneath the knees, separate the legs. This posture breaks up extensor patterns, controls excess flexion and, when used with a profiling bed, can mimic a sitting position for patients who do not have suitable seating (see Figure 10.1).

Low-friction sheets

Low-friction sheets, also known as slide sheets, are used to reposition a patient in bed, or to move them on to a shower trolley or lift bath trolley. The sheets are made of a durable, lightweight fabric that slides, rather than drags or lifts, a patient. This elimi-

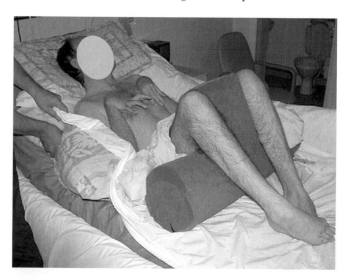

Figure 10.1 Positioning with T-roll (reproduced with permission from Priory Healthcare).

nates friction at the contact points between the individual and the bed and makes repositioning easier for both patient and nurse. The sheets are available in different sizes, are inexpensive and are easily cleaned and stored.

Cushions and padding

Pressure-reducing foam and gel cushions are available in a wide range of shapes and sizes and have similar conforming and supportive properties to those of the conforming mattresses (see Figure 10.2). They can be used to protect and support the buttocks and sacrum and can be supplied in different shapes and sizes to help position a person in a bed or chair, thus conferring a sense of security as well as giving support. Each patient's needs should be individually assessed in choosing the appropriate cushions and padding (McPeak 2000; Collins 2001; Khoulawa 2001; Cullum *et al.* 2002; Disabled Living Foundation 2002; Nursey 2002).

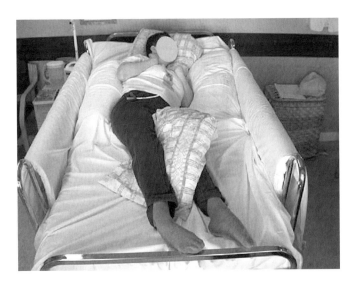

Figure 10.2 Positioning with sleep support (reproduced with permission from Priory Healthcare).

Patient hoists

A hoist can assist in many transfer tasks, such as lifting from bed, chair or floor, toileting or bathing, with the patient being supported in a semi-reclined position. The support can reduce the incidence of spasms and, if used properly, can confer a sense of safety that reduces the muscle tone that fear might provoke. Before operating the hoist, each nurse and carer needs to be confident in the way it moves, how it is operated and how to attach each sling safely and securely (Clevely 1996; Berg 1998; Busse 2000; Steed and Tracey 2000; Baptiste *et al.* 2002; Collins 2002).

Slings for hoists

The hoist should be compatible with different types of slings, so that the right sling can be used for each patient and purpose (Hall 2001; Medical Devices Agency 2003). Contoured head and body support slings are available in different sizes and include:

- a toileting sling with head support;
- a mesh sling for bathing and showering;
- a padded sling for general transfers and comfort.

Wheelchair seating

In seating a patient in a wheelchair the following criteria need to be met (Batavia 1998; Ham *et al.* 1998; White 1999; Collins 2001):

- manage trunk control;
- stabilise the hips;
- lift the head, enabling patients to make eye contact;
- offer shoulder support;
- be at the right height from knee to foot and correct thigh length;
- foot plates need to promote plantegrade flexion;
- give suitable cushioning to enhance tissue viability;
- have a tilt-in-space facility.

If a patient is seated well in a wheelchair that supports a good sitting posture they can gain several important benefits (see Figure 10.3). The chairs can have a tilt-in-space facility, which maintains the 90 degree angle of the hips to the trunk and over-

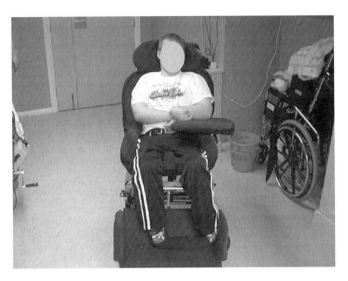

Figure 10.3 Seated in customised wheelchair (reproduced with permission from Priory Healthcare).

comes the effect of gravity as the patient tries to maintain a sitting posture against gravity. The good posture has several benefits, including stimulation of interaction through better eye contact, better swallowing, better lung function and capacity, improved gravitational pull and urine output, and sensory stimulation of feet giving sense of place and orientation in space.

Chairs

An ordinary bedside chair, which is often found in hospital settings, can cause serious postural problems as patients strive to maintain sitting balance against an unsuitable base of support. Electrically or manually operated chairs can have a tilt-in-space facility that gives much better support, postural balance and a greater sense of security (see Figure 10.4).

Walking aids such as sticks, frames and rolators

Patients need to be assessed as able to use these aids since some may produce unwanted movement patterns.

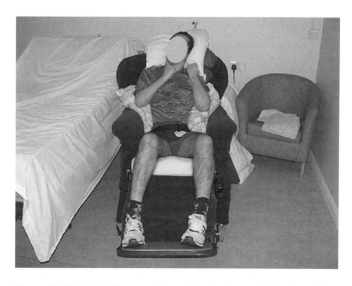

Figure 10.4 Seated with support (reproduced with permission from Priory Healthcare).

FRED'S CASE

Mobility and independence for Fred (see case study in the section on How to Use this Book) will depend on how far nurses are able to assist or help him plan his abilities to coincide with his times of optimum drug effect. However, he will need to understand that the reduction of his medication which is needed to try to clear up his hallucinations will probably reduce his mobility. In addition to a moving and handling assessment, nurses need to be guided by a physiotherapy assessment on safe and effective mobility aids that Fred can use. He will need good support to maintain a good seating posture, and a profiling bed will help. Exercise is important however, for his blood and for prevention of chest complications and pressure sores, and Fred will need assistance and encouragement to help him keep these benefits. It may help to use triggers to initiate movement such as a rocking rhythm and count-in when he is moving from one position to another or is walking. An adjustable-height bed or raiser chair set high when he is getting up will reduce effort and give him more stability. He can be encouraged to maintain dexterity and manipulation with games or hobby activity.

IRENE'S CASE

For Irene (see case study in the section How to Use this Book), transferring from bed to chair, toilet and bath may have become a problem made worse by fatigue and breathing difficulty. An adjustable-height bed with a profiling facility, and a chair that gives good postural support will support her trunk and help the dyspnoea due to impaired respiratory muscles. Slide sheets, hoists and other moving and handling equipment such as lift bath trolley may be needed, or eventually an electronic wheelchair. The disease seems to have progressed rapidly for Irene and the psychological impact of having to accept adaptive equipment or hoists can be deeply distressing. The emphasis needs to be on the maintenance of independence and on how a hoist can assist her to carry out meaningful activities in her life. The care team also need to be alert to the rapidity with which she may develop the need for other aids and adaptations. She may also get pain from muscle spasticity and cramps that may be helped by positioning, arm supports and medication.

NURSING ASSESSMENT

A thorough assessment of this activity should be done in conjunction with interdisciplinary team, taking into account the therapeutic approaches taken by the physiotherapist and occupational therapist to manage the physical symptoms of:

- tone;
- spasticity;
- posture;
- joint flexion, extension and range of movement;
- contracture;
- muscle weakness, flaccidity or floppiness, balance, incoordination and compensatory movement strategies (Edwards 2002). Miriam (see case study in the section on How to Use this Book) may still be recovering from a condition known as critical-illness neuropathy, which may occur in any patient who has spent some time in intensive care.

In addition, the occupational therapist will take into account how perceptual or cognitive impairments affect mobility (see Table 10.2). These include impairments of attention, memory, action planning and sequencing, space perception and other disturbances of visual perception (Grieve 1993).

Table 10.2 Mobility problems in different conditions.

	Possible motor impairments	Other factors affecting mobility
Acquired brain injury	Hemiplegia, hypotonicity, hyper tonicity, spasticity, flaccidity, ataxia, perseveration, tendonitis, impaired senses of balance and equilibrium, loss of proprioception	Visual field deficits, double vision, body image disturbance, body awareness deficit, neglect, dysphasia
Multiple sclerosis	Ataxia, tremor, fatigue, spasticity, incoordination, loss of range of motion, contractures, impaired balance	Pain, cognitive impairment, depression, dysphasia, urinary frequency and urgency
Parkinson's disease	Resting tremor, decreased movements (bradykinesia) rigidity, decreased facial expression, decreased blinking, shuffling gait	Side effects of drug treatments: hypotension, visual hallucination, bladder retention, chorea (involuntary movements of face and extremities), dystonia, duskiness, on–off fluctuations from under- or overtreatment, confusion, pyschosis
Ataxia	Intention tremor, unsteady gait, tripping, stumbling overshooting the mark when reaching or stepping	May accompany brain tumour, stroke, multiple sclerosis, cerebellar haemorrhage, infarct tumour
Muscle weakness due to neuromuscular junction disorders	Fluctuating weakness that is symmetrical, facial muscle weakness, double vision. Swallowing and respiration may be affected	

Nursing assessment can be carried out while caring for the patient in many of the activities of living, in conjunction with the overall assessment outlined in Chapter 2, and could include the following areas (Nieuwenhaus 1993; Jones 1999; Barnes and Ward 2000; Kirrane 2000; Hollerbach 2001; Edwards 2002):

- In what way does the person respond to sensory stimulation such as sight, sound, smell and touch?
- Does the sensation trigger spasms, spasticity or unwanted compensatory movements?
- Is there a sensation that the patient relies on to trigger a movement pattern? For example, is movement prompted by guiding the limb or using the key points of control.
- Is movement prompted by giving simple step-by-step verbal instructions? Is movement prompted by a rhythmic lead such as a counted rocking and one-two-three?
- Are there any dyskinesias, or slow writhing involuntary movements or other special problems such as on–off periods in patients who have Parkinson's disease? Does this mean that the medication may need reviewing?
- Is there a physiotherapy assessment that sets out moving, handling, positioning, pressure-relieving and mobilising strategies?
- If not, is referral to a physiotherapist indicated by evidence of abnormal tone and position, such as slumping or leaning over to one side, balance reactions, extension, flexion, range of movement, spasticity or contracture?
- Does the act of mobilising cause excessive fatigue?
- Are there occupational therapy guidelines on how to assist the patient in improving attention, memory, action planning and sequencing through the activity of mobilising?
- What safety factors need to be considered in relation to staff, patient and carers?
- What equipment and resources are needed, and do these need to be ordered, purchased, hired, borrowed?
- Have employer policies on risk assessment been carried out correctly?
- Are there any staff/carer/patient education or training needs? Good teamwork, ongoing assessment and interdisci-

plinary planning are essential if all of the patient's needs are to be met.

INTERVENTIONS

The main goals of intervention are: to maintain good posture; to correct balance mechanism; to maintain soft tissue condition; to improve tone, mobility, symmetry and balance; to reduce complications; and to make efficient use of energy. The following can all help to achieve these goals:

- A gentle and calming approach will help relax muscles. Fear can increase muscle tone considerably and pain.
- Use appropriate moving and handling equipment, giving the patient clear, paced guidance.
- Hand over control to patients whenever possible, for example by allowing them to operate the hoist switch. The advance organisers and a degree of control give patients the chance to use anticipatory systems and can help prevent muscle tone from increasing owing to fear.
- Choose the most appropriate mattress. Airflow mattresses or water mattresses may be unsuitable because they increase tone and inhibit movement. Individuals differ according to their patterns and their response to neurological damage and specialist help may be needed.
- Use a four-section profiling bed and change position as agreed with the care team every two hours, taking into consideration other medical needs. For example, patients with a tracheostomy may need positioning to help drain secretions. Patients with gastrostomy feeding will need to be nursed at a 45 degree angle when fed to ensure the feed is tolerated.
- Use a T-roll to break up extensor patterns and prevent contractures in brain-injured patients. If a T-roll is not available, use a rolled up duvet, beanbags and pillows. This support prevents side-sweeping, scissoring and foot drop.
- When the patient is side lying, place padded protection between the knees which gives pressure relief all the way down to the ankles. Check that the shoulder is not trapped and that the upper arm is supported. This prevents the development of a painful shoulder and spasticity in the arm.

- Liaise with the physiotherapist about adopting an inhibitory position in which the patient needs to lie or sit, using special equipment if necessary.
- Maintain the head in a good midline position, well supported by pillows to help maintain body symmetry.
- Minimise noxious stimuli that can trigger spasticity. This includes managing the bowels, bladder and pain effectively. Unchecked spasticity is very painful and can lead to other problems such as skin deterioration.
- Control pain.
- Use active and passive exercises only if recommended by the physiotherapist. Range-of-motion exercises can be harmful if not done appropriately and correctly. Try different side lying, sitting and standing positions to help find the postures that most inhibit spasticity.
- Use splints and casts as appropriate. Splinting may be used to compensate for weak or absent muscle function or to resist the action of high muscle tone.
- Contact a specialist if seating or a sitting position is a problem. An ordinary armchair is not suitable if a person has no sitting balance. Abnormal patterns develop or skin integrity is compromised. A profiling bed may be the most suitable equipment in some circumstances to enable patients to assume a safe sitting position (Cullum *et al*. 2002; Edwards 2002).
- Evaluate motivation and develop a plan to help maintain it. Refer to the clinical psychologist if mood is low or disruptive and interfering with progress.

All of these factors will have been considered in developing a plan of care for Gary and Mark (see case studies in the section on How to Use this Book).

GARY'S CASE

If Gary's abnormal posture and muscle tone are unchecked, permanent contractures and permanent abnormality of posture may lead to several handicaps in other activities of living such as eating, drinking, watching television or engaging in interactions with others.

Muscle tone

The tone in his right arm and legs is likely to be high. The high tone is caused by lack of inhibition from motor centres in the brain, which normally modulate the high tone that is initiated in the spinal cord. This high tone in his arms needs to be controlled by the inhibitory positioning of the limb, possibly with the use of a soft splint, range-of-movement exercises and passive stretches. A profiling bed and/or a T-roll can help to break up spastic extensor patterns in his lower limbs.

Moving and handling

When moving and handling Gary, nurses can use the concept of key points of control to facilitate movement. The key points of control are points in the body that can unlock a movement pattern from the brain and spinal cord. They can be used in movement facilitation to help relearn good movement patterns and can be demonstrated by a physiotherapist.

Seating

A full assessment should identify the most suitable type of seating, such as a tilt-in-space chair, rather than a reclining chair. If Gary sits out in an ordinary armchair he risks having his head pulled further down on to his chest, as the antigravity muscles are weak, and these neck muscles will be unable to overcome gravity. He may also start to try using his stiff legs as a brake to stop him falling out of the chair, thereby further increasing unwanted tone in his body.

If suitable seating is not available then a positional programme of profiling bed positional change and limited periods of sitting out should be instigated. Risk assessment and a rationale for the posture management programme should be documented. Such postural management should prevent the development of pressure sores, chest infections and further problems of tone associated with lying in one position. This change of position is important because it changes the base of support and consequently the muscle tone distribution in the body.

Walking

When Gary is walking, the spasticity interferes with normal patterns of movement and his stability is reduced. It may be necessary to discourage him from independent walking until his muscle tone settles. Of course, if he has cognitive or language impairments, it may be difficult to get him to understand the need for limitation of his activity and to engage his co-operation.

MARK'S CASE

In developing Mark's plan of care, there may be a range of options and possible interventions. For example, there could be several reasons for his unsteady and uneven gait and his lolling to one side as he sits. These include hemiplegia, brain stem damage, damage to accoustic nerve or eardrum, dizziness, or loss of proprioception

If the TPR and BP readings are abnormal, they may indicate that the autonomic system is struggling to maintain homeostasis. The blood pressure may drop on standing or when exerting, or there may be cardiac arrhythmias which are contributing to unsteadiness and dizziness. The nurse should initiate a lying and standing blood pressure recording, and a pulse and apex recording. An ECG may be ordered. If there are abnormalities, refer to the physician, who may prescribe controlling medication.

If there is damage to the accoustic nerve, this may be causing dizziness. The nurse should refer to the physician, who may order an MRI scan that may show lesions on the accoustic nerve or brain stem. Brain stem auditory evoked potentials, which deliver click stimuli to either ear, may also be ordered. They may also show up damage in the auditory pathways.

Mark may have *ataxia*, a disorder of co-ordination, balance and rhythm that may be caused by damage to his cerebellum sustained in the fight. If ataxia is suspected, refer to the physiotherapist for a functional assessment.

He may have a *hemiparesis* and, while walking, will list towards the weaker side and bump into things. He may have visible muscle wasting on the weaker side, and there would be asymmetry in the limb power estimations that form part of the nursing neurological assessment. He may easily fatigue while sitting and loll as a way of trying to rest and sleep. He may have damage to cranial and spinal nerves that weakens the control of his head and neck muscles. If any of these are suspected, Mark should be referred to the physiotherapist for evaluation of sitting balance, trunk control, proprioception and muscle fatigue when sitting and walking.

He may have a *visual disturbance*, such as double vision (diplopia) or have only half his visual field (hemianopia). This would mean he would not see objects on the affected side. If he has restricted or weakened head movements, he may be unable to compensate for this. If visual disturbance is suspected, Mark should be referred to the physician who would carry out a visual field and acuity assessment and may order an investigation of Mark's visually evoked potentials.

SUMMARY

❏ Normal movement develops as patterns of movement become automatic.

❏ Postural tone is the muscle tone generated by nerve stimulation to allow muscle to relax and contract in patterns. The key points of control can be used to unlock patterns that may have been lost and the base of support needs to be taken into account in all tone management strategies.

❏ Spasticity is excessive muscle tone that causes pain and abnormal limb position, interfering with independence. It can be managed by using inhibitory positioning, removing triggers, and by using suitable antispasmodics. Uncorrected it can lead to contracture, tendon shortening and atrophied muscles.

❏ The general principles in managing hemiplegia lie in understanding the flaccid or spastic nature of the hemiplegia, liaising with other team members to ensure the position in bed, the transfers from the bed and the seating arrangements are therapeutic for that patient.

❏ Selection of equipment such as hoists, wheelchairs, tilt-in-space chairs profiling beds, cushions and mattresses must be made on clinical reasoning of the costs and benefits to the patients in promoting comfort and preventing complications.

❏ Nursing assessment and care planning need to be developed closely with the multidisciplinary team, taking into account the patient's additional sensory, cognitive or perceptual problems and the need to help them develop maximum safe independence.

REFERENCES

Ada, L. and O'Dwyer, M. (2001) Do associated reactions in the upper limb after stroke contribute to contracture formation? *Clinical Rehabilitation* **15** (2), 186–94.

Atwood, R. M. (1999) Managing contractures in a long term setting. *OT Practice* **4** (4), 20–5.

Baptiste, A., Tiesman, H., Nelso, A. and Lloyd, J. (2002) Current issues: technology to reduce nurse back injuries. *Rehabilitation Nursing* **27** (2), 43–4.

Barnes, M. P. and Johnson, G. R. (2001) *Upper Motor Neurone Syndrome and Spasticity: Clinical Management and Neurophysiology*. Cambridge University Press, Cambridge.

Barnes, M. P. and Ward, A. B. (2000) *Textbook of Rehabilitation Medicine*. Oxford University Press, Oxford.

Batavia, M. (1998) *The Wheelchair Evaluation Guide*. Butterworth-Heinemann, New York.

Berg, V. J. (1998) *Ergonomics in Health Care and Rehabilitation*. Butterworth-Heinemann, New York.

Busse, M. (2000) Effective rehabilitation and hoisting equipment: a case study. *Nursing and Residential Care* **2** (4), 168–73.

Carr, J. H. and Shepherd, D. (1998) *Neurological Rehabilitation: Optimising Motor Performance*. Butterworth-Heinemann, Oxford.

Clevely, R. C. (1996) *Hoist Lifts and Transfers*. Disability Information Trust, Oxford.

Collins, F. (2001) Sitting-pressure ulcer development. *Nursing Standard* **15** (22), 54–6.

Collins, F. (2002) Selecting the most appropriate hoist for residential settings. *Nursing and Residential Care* **4** (5), 222–4, 226–7, 244–5.

Cullum, N., Deeks, J., Sheldon, T. A., Song, F. and Fletcher, A. W. (2002) Beds mattresses and cushions for pressure sore prevention and treatment. *The Cochrane Library*, Issue 1, Update Software, Oxford.

Disabled Living Foundation (2002) Properties and features of a pressure relief mattresses or beds, available at http://www.dlf.org.uk

Dressler, D. (2000) *Botulinum Toxin Therapy*. Thieme, Stuggart.

Edwards, S. (2002) *Neurological Physiotherapy*, 2nd edn. Churchill Livingstone, Edinburgh.

Elovic, E. and Zafonte, R. D. (2001) Spasticity management in traumatic brain injury. *Physical Medicine and Rehabilitation State of the Art Reviews* **15** (2), 327–48.

Gracies, J. M., Nance, P., Elovic, E., McGuire, J. and Simpson, J. (1997) Traditional pharmacological treatments for spasticity. Part II: General and regional Treatments. In Kimiura, J. (ed.), *Spasticity: Aetiology, Evalaution and management. Muscle and Nerve,* Supplement 6.

Gray, B., Delve, M. and Robinson, F. (1997) Out to tender: the nurse's role in awarding the contract for therapeutic bed/mattress hire. *Journal of Nursing Management* **5** (4), 217–22.

Grieve, J. (1993) *Neuropsychology for Occupational Therapists.* Blackwell Science, Oxford.

Grissom, S. P. and Blanton, S. (2001) Treatment of upper motorneurone plantar flexion by using an adjustable ankle–foot orthosis. *Archives of Physical Medicine and Rehabilitation* **82** (2), 270–3.

Hall, D. (2001) Risk assessment of the compatability of hoists and slings. *British Journal of Therapy and Rehabilitation* **8** (12), 472, 474–5.

Ham, R., Aldersea, P. and Porter, D. (1998) *Wheelchair Users and Postural Seating: A Clinical Approach.* Churchill Livingstone, Edinburgh.

Hampton, S. (1998) Can electric beds aid pressure sore prevention in hospitals? *British Journal of Nursing* **7** (17), 1010–17.

Hannah, M. (1995) *Rehabilitation for the Neurological Patient.* Churchill Livingstone, Edinburgh.

Harding, P. (2001) Early management of spasticity in patients with acute acquired brain injury. *Physiotherapy* **87** (1), 25–9.

Hartshorn, J. C. (2001) Abrupt alterations in mobility. In Stewart-Amidei, C. and Kunkel, J. A. (eds), *AANN's Neuroscience Nursing.* W. B. Saunders, Philadelphia, chapter 20.

Harvey, L. A. and Herbert, R. D. (2002) Muscle stretching for treatment and prevention of contracture in people with spinal cord injury. *Spinal Cord* **40** (1), 1–9.

Harvey, L. A., Herbert, R. D. and Crosbie, J. (2002) Does stretching induce lasting increases in joint ROM? a systematic review. *Physiotherapy Research International* **7** (1), 1–13.

Hollerbach, A. D. (2001) Assessment of human mobility. In Stewart-Amidei, C. and Kunkel, J. A. (eds), *AANN's Neuroscience Nursing.* W. B. Saunders, Philadelphia, chapter 19.

Johnstone, M. (1991) *Therapy for Stroke.* Churchill Livingstone, Edinburgh.

Johnstone, M. (1995) *Restoration of Normal Movement after Stroke.* Churchill Livingstone, Edinburgh.

Jones, M. (1999) Preventing contractures. *Nursing* **29** (10), 10.

Kamensek, J. (1999a) Continuous intrathecal baclofen infusions: an introduction and overview. *Axone* **20** (3), 67–72.

Kamensek, J. (1999b) Continuous intrathecal baclofen infusions: an introduction and overview. *Axone* **20** (4), 93–8.

Khoulawa, J. (2001) Product focus: Esprit HR mattress cover in pressure ulcer formation. *British Journal of Nursing* **19** (16), 1073–4.

Kilbride, C. and McDonnell, A. (2000) Spasticity: the role of physiotherapy. *British Journal of Therapy and Rehabilitation* **7** (2), 61–4.

Kirker, S. G. B., Jenner, J. R., Simpson, D. S. and Wing, A. M. (2000) Changing patterns of postural hip muscle activity during recovery from stroke. *Clinical Rehabilitation* **14** (6), 618–26.

Kirrane, C. (2000) Evidence-based practice in neurology: a team approach to development. *Nursing Standard* **14** (52), 43–5.

Lynch, M. and Grisogono, V. (1991) *Strokes and Head Injuries: A Guide for Patients Families, Friends and Carers*. John Murray, London.

McPeak, L. (2000) Beds, mattresses, lifters, and lift chairs: practical considerations. *Physical Medicine and Rehabilitation State of the Art Reviews* **14** (3), 493–514.

Medical Devices Agency (2003) Evaluations of equipment to assist moving and handling people, available at http://www.medical-devices.gov.uk/mda

Mitchell, J., Jones, J. and McNair, B. (1998) *Choosing Beds for Hospitals*. King's Fund, London.

Nieuwenhaus, R. (1993) *Teamwork in Neurology*. Chapman & Hall, London.

Nursey, M. (2002) Product focus: Swift and clean – setting new standards in equipment design. *British Journal of Therapy and Rehabilitation* **9** (10), 409–10.

O'Connor, H. (2000) Decontaminating beds and mattresses. *NTplus* **96** (46), 2, 4–5.

Perry, J. (1999) The use of gait analysis for surgical recommendations in traumatic brain injury. *Journal of Head Trauma Rehabilitation* **14** (2), 116–35.

Pollock, A. S., Durward, B. R. and Rowe, P. J. (2000) What is balance? *Clinical Rehabilitation* 402–6.

Porter, B. (2001) Nursing management of spasticity. *Primary Health Care* **11** (1), 25–7.

Reed, K. L. (2001) Quick Reference to Occupational Therapy 2nd ed. Aspen Maryland.

Rithalia, S. and Kenney, L. (2000) Mattresses and beds: reducing and relieving pressure. *Nursing Times* **96** (36), 9–10.

Russell, L. (2001) Tissue viability: overview of research to investigate pressure reducing surfaces. *British Journal of Nursing* **10** (21), 1421–6.

Rutishauser, S. (1994) *Physiology and Anatomy: A Basis for Nursing and Healthcare*. Churchill Livingstone, Edinburgh.

Steed, R. and Tracey, C. (2000) Equipment for moving and handling. *British Journal of Therapy and Rehabilitation* **7** (10), 430–5.

Stockmann, T. (2001) Casting for the person with spasticity. *Topics in Stroke Rehabilitation* **8** (1), 27–35.

Sullivan, M. (2000) Positioning of patients with severe traumatic brain injury – research based practice. *Journal of Neuroscience Nursing* **20**, 223–8.

Taricco, M., Adone, R., Pagliacci, C. and Telaro, E. (2003) Pharmacological interventions for spasticity following spinal cord injury (Cochrane Review). *The Cochrane Library*, Issue 1, Update Software, Oxford.

Turner-Stokes, L. and Ward, A. (2002) Botulinum toxin in the management of spasticity in adults. *Clinical Medicine* **2** (2), 127–30.

Wallen, M. (1995) An evaluation of the soft splint in the acute management of elbow hypertonicity. *Occupational Therapy Journal of Research* **15** (1), 3–15.

Watkins, C. A. (1999) Mechanical and neurophysiological changes in spastic muscles: serial casting in spastic equinovarus following traumatic brain injury. *Physiotherapy* **85** (11), 603–9.

White, E. A. (1999) Wheelchair cushions: assessment and prescription. *British Journal of Therapy and Rehabilitation* **6** (2), 75–81.

Working and Playing

11

INTRODUCTION

Working and playing give us a sense of being part of a wider community and social belonging, a sense of achievement, the chance to feel satisfaction at being able express creativity and to feel successful in problem solving as well as (in the case of work) the obvious practical benefit of an income to support our needs and desires (Cantrell 1997). Neurological impairments often adversely affect a person's role in the family, among friends and in the community, although there are many support groups, charity and self-help groups that exemplify how a positive attitude and determination to take advantage of opportunities can support an excellent quality of life despite having to give up work or switch to a different job.

Eye–hand–mind integration gives a powerful sense of competence and satisfies the need to achieve mastery, efficacy and autonomy. Many patients with a disability say that the disability influences the quality of their lives and their sense of well-being (Pedretti and Early 1996). The sense of well-being can be threatened not only by disability but also by a preoccupation with the negative and with disability that can lead to serious underestimation of ability either by the person themself or by others.

This chapter outlines the important role of mood and attitude in coming to terms with neurological impairments. It also differentiates aspects of assessing cognitive and perceptual deficit and ability, and describes the strategies that people can use to compensate or retrain. Fatigue and depression are also outlined as a common feature of neurological conditions and the ways in which the effects on quality of life can be minimised.

LEARNING OBJECTIVES
❏ Discuss the influence of neurological impairment on mood and motivation.
❏ Differentiate among a range of cognitive and perceptual disturbances affecting memory, attention, sequencing, visual perception of depth, figure/ground discrimination, object recognition, spatial orientation and language disturbance.
❏ Appreciate importance of collaborative care planning with occupational therapists in minimising fatigue and using daily activities to help with cognitive and perceptual retraining.
❏ Discuss the importance of giving information to patient and family and identifying support networks to motivate the recovery and rehabilitation process.
❏ Outline support and information available at government level on disability.

INFLUENCE OF NEUROLOGICAL IMPAIRMENT ON MOOD AND MOTIVATION
The realisation of disability may produce disturbing thoughts and feelings such as disbelief, denial, anger, panic, self-devaluation and guilt, which may swing over to hope and encouragement, feelings of being comforted and of relief, that gradually approach acceptance. The impairments that people are likely to experience as disabling or handicapping include those that are obvious to others such as hemiplegia, aphasia, dysarthria. However, those which are less visible but of which the person themself may be acutely aware, such as bowel or bladder disturbance, can inhibit social life. In addition, some perceptual and cognitive deficits may become evident only during conversation or while carrying out a job. These subtler impairments cause loss of confidence and reluctance to engage in social interaction and community life, and depression may develop.

ROLE OF OCCUPATIONAL THERAPISTS
Engaging in activities and occupations involves the whole human being in the development of the skill. It requires sub-

routines such as planning, problem solving, application of work habits, knowing and following rules, identifying and correcting mistakes. Occupational therapists are skilled in using standardised test batteries and functional activities to assess a person's physical, perceptual, cognitive and behavioural attributes. They can identify the practical implications of the deficits identified in the tests. Areas of strength and weakness can be deduced and potential treatment approaches identified. Activation of interests through occupation is a way of tapping into the intrinsic motivation that will energise the person not only for the short term but also for life in the real world of the home and the community.

The main standardised tests include:

- Rivermead Perceptual Assessment Battery (RPAB);
- Chessington Occupational Therapy Neurological Assessment Battery (COTNAB);
- Rivermead Behavioural Memory Battery;
- Behavioural Inattention Test (BIT).

Using these tests and observations of patients, occupational therapists can liaise with nurses in producing activity analyses for everyday tasks such as brushing one's teeth or buying a newspaper. The analysis highlights the perceptual, cognitive and physical capacities required to carry out the activity. From this a therapeutic programme can be developed for individuals according to their abilities and deficits, which nurses can incorporate in their daily care (Grieve 1993).

COGNITIVE DEFICITS

Cognitive disorders due to brain damage from neurological degeneration or trauma alter a person's experiences and responses to stimuli and may manifest as attention, orientation or concentration problems.

Different levels of cognitive deficit (Table 11.1) can affect aspects of a person's work and leisure life in the following ways:

Table 11.1 A classification of cognitive deficits (adapted from Edmans *et al.* 2001).

Classification	Attention	Visual processing	Memory	Information processing	Executive functions
Input	Focused	Visual cognition	Sensory memory	Classification of received information	Self-awareness
Storage	Sustained	Spatial problem	Long-term memory		Goal setting
Processing	Selective	Alexia	Short-term memory	Memory	Self-initiation
Output	Alternating	Figure/ground	Storage	Organisational skills:	Self-inhibition
		Position in space	Retrieval	separating	Planning
		Constructional problems		closing	Self-monitoring
		Contextual clues to gain meaning for an image		combining	Flexible problem solving
		Visual memory		sorting	
		Pattern recognition:		ranking	
		Colour		sequencing	
		Shape		categorising	
		Contour		grouping	
		Texture			
		Details			
		Scanning			
		Visual attention			
		Oculomotor skills			
		Visual field			
		Visual acuity			

- Memory loss can make daily life and ordinary basic activities difficult and makes learning new skills very effortful.
- Reasoning and judgement, problem solving and behavioural regulation may be impaired but may not be obvious.
- The speed of information processing may be altered, making it difficult to deal with information coming from different directions and sources.
- Attention and concentration lapses can cause problems when attention needs to be divided between two tasks.
- Visuo-spatial perception is also sometimes impaired.
- Some medications for pain, fatigue or depression may cause cognitive deficits.

The aim of intervention is to use prompts and triggers to help overcome deficits and to engender a positive attitude.

Therapeutic objectives
- Maintain independence as far as possible.
- Achieve stability and reliability as a member of the community.
- Develop the capacity and potential to contribute to society.

Therapeutic approaches

- A retraining approach, where progressively more challenging exercises incrementally strengthen impaired function. Behaviour modification techniques can help people relearn tasks with fixed sequences of steps, such as washing and dressing. The techniques use:
  - praise to reinforce desired behaviours, and
  - ignoring the client so that no reinforcement follows an undesired behaviour (Reed 2001).
- Verbal mediation to control behaviour through self-instruction and self-regulation.
- Using prompts and triggers to compensate for deficit. These might include:
  - a large page-a-day diary and routines of consulting it;
  - establishment of a fixed routine, such as always keeping things in the same place, to help establish a motor routine;

- doing only one thing at a time and removing background noise and distractions;
- admitting to a memory problem;
- using visual imagery, since a mental picture can consolidate information;
- use of technology such as Dictaphones, bleepers, timers, alarms etc.

PERCEPTUAL DEFICITS

Perceptual deficits can be difficult to distinguish from cognitive deficits, and it is important to consider these as well as other impairments that may affect performance. Perceptual deficits include:

- *Body image*. The person may lack the visual and mental image of the body.
- *Body scheme*. The deficit is a difficulty in perceiving one's body parts in relation to each other and in relation to how to move oneself.
- *Spatial relations deficit*. Shows up as a difficulty perceiving the position of two objects in relation to each other (up, across, over, on etc.). It affects the ability to distinguish an object from its background, the difference between a cup and a jug, difficulty in route finding and difficulty in judging depth and distance.
- *Agnosia*. This is a deficit in interpreting objects perceived by the senses. It can include difficulty in recognising people, faces, possessions, colours, the feel of objects, differentiating between sounds.

Therapeutic approaches

Occupational therapists can design specific tasks and programmes based on formal assessment to help overcome perceptual deficits. This would typically involve the following (Edmans *et al.* 2001):

- Beginning with simple tasks and graduate to more complex ones.
- Using demonstration, imitation or gesture to facilitate the activity.

- Deciding whether to use verbal or written instructions, or both.
- Using repetition and practice.
- Reinforcing positive behaviours.
- Breaking down tasks into stages.
- Developing a systematic pattern and routines.
- Ensuring constancy in the approach and method of treatment by the whole team.

Body image and scheme deficits

Approaches that can help to make the person more aware of parts of the body and how to carry out activities that involve them include the following (Edmans *et al.* 2001):

- Encouraging the person to name the parts and position of the body during activities such as washing and dressing.
- Assembling, drawing and dressing human-shaped models.
- Stimulating awareness of neglect of a body side or part by approaching from that side, and by increasing attention to that part or side by drawing attention to environmental landmarks.
- Drawing and copying objects; games that require scanning a visual field such as cards, dominoes.
- Using activities of living to raise awareness in placing and positioning objects.

Spatial relations

Activities that can help the person develop more awareness of the relationship between objects, distinguish foreground from background, depth and distance include the following (Edmans *et al.* 2001):

- Use opportunities that arise to help the person find items against a similar or contrasting background.
- Use domino-type games, hidden objects in a picture.
- Ask person to trace around the outline of an object.
- Use three-dimensional block-and-cube design and copying tasks, and name the shapes.
- Encourage person to verbalise relationships of items to themselves: in front/behind/above/to my left.
- Use opportunities in living activities to practise identifying shapes, relationships, foreground and background.

Agnosia
- Use opportunities to help the person recognise differences and similarities between objects, starting with very different objects and gradually working towards objects that are more similar.
- Give matching tasks such as numbers, colours, symmetrical and reversed shapes. Use pictures and three-dimensional blocks.
- Spot-the-difference type puzzles.
- Use everyday opportunities to help the person distinguish differences in form, shape and colours, feel and texture, and sounds such as a car engine and lawn mower.

FATIGUE

Fatigue is an overwhelming sense of tiredness, lack of energy and feeling of exhaustion that is characteristically severe. It is sometimes difficult to distinguish this from limb weakness or depression (see Table 11.2). It can appear as laziness, or it may appear as a worsening of cognitive function, mobility or muscle spasms. It is associated with a range of neurological impairments and conditions, and particularly with multiple sclerosis.

Primary fatigue
Primary fatigue is a direct result of damage to the central nervous system as the body responds by slowing down reactions and thus causing fatigue. People with neurological problems may experience different types of fatigue (Multiple Sclerosis Society 2001):

- *Lassitude* an overwhelming tiredness not directly related to participation in activity or exercise.
- *'Short circuiting' fatigue* which occurs in specific muscle groups, for example the hand after writing for a while.
- *Heat sensitivity fatigue*, which may occur because of climate and seasonal change or following heat-producing activity such as hot baths or hot meals.

Secondary fatigue
Secondary fatigue is caused by factors other than neurological damage (Multiple Sclerosis Society 2001):

Table 11.2 Assessment of the person with fatigue (Burgess 2002).

Assess	Rationale for assessment	Action
Sleeping pattern	Disturbed sleep will exacerbate fatigue	Determine cause of poor sleep and liaise with appropriate interdisciplinary team member
Temperature and pulse	If infection present fatigue will be worse than usual	If temperature elevated, liaise with doctor and administer any medication as prescribed
Send MSU for culture	People with MS are often vulnerable to urine infections	If positive, liaise with doctor and treat appropriately
Normal activity patterns	Is patient too sedentary or too active, have activity levels changed	Liaise with occupational therapist and physiotherapist and advise patient appropriately
Pattern of fatigue	Are there any exacerbating factors, e.g. hot baths?	Check patient's understanding of triggers and advise accordingly
Current medication	Some medications can cause drowsiness	Liaise with doctor if there are any concerns
Fluid balance	Patient may have frequency and/or nocturia which disturbs their sleep and causes many trips to the toilet during the day, increasing energy expenditure	Maintain accurate fluid balance, encourage patient to drink $1-1\frac{1}{2}$ litres fluid daily. Ensure ready access to toilet when required. Liaise with appropriate member of interdisciplinary team re bladder symptoms/access to toilet etc.
Mood	Low mood may be caused by fatigue or may be an exacerbating factor	Ensure patient has opportunity to voice concerns. Liaise with appropriate members of interdisciplinary team as necessary
Patient's understanding of fatigue	Patient may not be employing appropriate self-help strategies	Educate patient re cause and management of fatigue, refer to occupational therapist and/or physiotherapy as appropriate
Understanding of patient's family/ friends etc.	Others may have unrealistic expectations of the person with MS	Educate appropriate individuals re cause and nature of fatigue
Aids and adaptations used at home/work	Lack of appropriate aids and adaptations may cause unnecessary energy expenditure	Refer to occupational therapist

- *Sleep disturbance* that may be caused by spasms, pain, urinary urgency at night, depression or anxiety.
- *Infection* may cause the body temperature to rise.
- *Exertion* – the increased effort of maintaining balance and co-ordination can cause fatigue.
- *Medications* such as baclofen and diazepam may cause tiredness or drowsiness as a side effect.
- *Depression* may be due to nerve damage or because of the emotional impact of adjusting to neurological damage and chronic illness or disability.
- *Environmental factors* such as the lighting and the temperature may cause fatigue because of increased straining or because the heat exacerbates fatigue.

Possible triggers of secondary fatigue may include:

- environmental factors such as hot and humid climate, a hot bath, raised body temperature, highly spiced food or an infection;
- poor diet or eating too little or too much;
- overexertion without rest periods;
- stressful and emotional situations.

Fatigue management

Fatigue management programmes involve looking at how an activity can be simplified and at a range of labour-saving devices.

- Ensure a balance between activity and rest.
- Discussion and consultation with the occupational therapist and physiotherapist on: timing and scheduling of treatments; activity analysis to develop energy-efficient strategies; exercises that improve not only muscle stretch and strength but also circulation and aerobic function; and relaxation and rest techniques.
- The importance of prioritising and planning ahead. Making a list will show what is obviously a priority, what can be shared, altered or eliminated. Essential jobs can then be properly planned.
- Keeping some flexibility about routine to take into account the body's fatigue levels.

- Administration of amantidine or other drug such as modafinil. These can be used to treat primary fatigue. Although they may be effective in managing the fatigue, they may also produce side effects such as dizziness, headache and difficulty sleeping.
- Review of drugs that may be causing fatigue.
- Diet and nutrition have an important role here as well as other lifestyle habits such as alcohol intake or cigarette smoking.

IRENE'S CASE

Irene (see case study in the section on How to Use this Book) may well benefit from assessment by an occupational therapist to help her develop work-simplification and energy-conserving tactics such as mechanical aids, electronic aids, adapted utensils and equipment, electronic environmental controls and adaptations to her home living environment.

LOUISE'S CASE

Louise (see case study in the section on How to Use this Book) will probably experience fatigue and from many contributory factors in addition to the effect of demyelination (Burgess 2002). A thorough assessment will help manage and identify the contributory factors. The care planning needs to be negotiated with Louise and the interdisciplinary team to ensure that test, investigations and treatments are spread throughout the day to allow time for rest. A number of advisory leaflets are available from the Multiple Sclerosis Society that give practical tips on energy conservation and self-help. Louise is clearly under a lot of stress and is low in mood, which will be exacerbating her fatigue.

DEPRESSION

Depression may be a normal part of the grieving process and coming to terms with disability. This grieving process is discussed more fully in Chapter 14. Depressed mood needs to be distinguished from major depression since the latter can be extremely serious. Possible indicators of depression are set out in Table 11.3. The Multiple Sclerosis Society suggests using the acronym SIGE CAPS to explore a person's low mood:

Table 11.3 Possible indicators of depression.

Physical	Psychological
Poor appetite	Negative thoughts
Weight loss	Black and white all-or nothing thinking
Increased appetite and weight gain	Loss of interest or pleasure
Altered sleep pattern, particularly early morning wakening	Indecisiveness and poor concentration
Excessive dream sleep	Preoocuaption with certain ideas and thoughts
Lethargy or agitation	Self-blame and guilt

- *Sleep.* Is there a change in your sleep pattern?
- *Interest.* Have you noticed you are less interested in things that typically gave you pleasure?
- *Guilt.* Do you think you are more guilty or remorseful than usual about things you have either done or not done?
- *Energy.* Has there been a change in your energy levels lately?
- *Concentration.* Do you find your memory or concentration less sharp than usual?
- *Appetite.* Has your appetite changed recently?
- *Psychomotor.* Does the patient exhibit motor retardation or agitation?
- *Suicide.* Have you thought of ending your life? This is an important question. People who tell you how they might commit suicide can be dangerously depressed (Griffin and Tyrell 2003).

If a nurse suspects that a patient may be depressed, these features should be explored sensitively in a quiet and un-interrupted environment. The role of the nurse depends on their level of experience and expertise in counselling. These skills may help alleviate fears and concerns in milder forms of depression, but if the depression is more severe the assistance of a qualified counsellor or psychologist will probably be needed.

Treatment (Griffin and Tyrell 2003)

- *Drug therapy* should be the first line of treatment if the depression is severe, as long as the patient wants it. This would probably be a selective serotonin re-uptake inhibitor.
- *Psychotherapy* should be considered the first line of treatment if the depression is mild to moderate, if it is non-psychotic, not chronic, not highly recurrent and the patient wants it. It should identify the cause and attempt to alter negative thinking patterns to a more positive thinking style.
- It is also worth remembering that *support groups* can provide a valuable source of peer support.

Depression is common after stroke (RCP 1999) in people who have multiple sclerosis (Stuifbergen and Rogers 1997), and occurring in as many as 50% of patients with Parkinson's disease (Calne and Kumar 2003). It is often difficult to differentiate severe depression in people who have these neurological impairments from the symptoms of neuronal damage itself. Since depression can have such a deleterious effect on recovery, rehabilitation and lifestyle, it must be assumed to be a constant threat to well-being and included as part of ongoing assessment.

ELLA'S CASE

The distress that Ella (see case study in the section on How to Use this Book) experiences may be related to pain and in addition may be an expression of a catastrophic response to what has happened to her. This is a profound emotional and psychological disturbance as realisation takes place of the enormity of what has happened, and is experienced as an overwhelming sense of fear, anxiety, hopelessness, frustration, loss and grief. Her depression may also be caused by damage to neural tissue from the stroke, and stroke patients, in common with people who have other neurological conditions, may experience emotional lability. Any strategies a nurse can think to provide emotional support, reassurance and information should be explored to help Ella through this difficult time and may involve family, friends, volunteers and contact with a person who has gone through a similar experience and can offer support and encouragement.

Table 11.4 Factors which affect families adaptation efforts.

Positive factors	Negative factors
Adequate financial resources	Continuous and unremitting anger over disease
Adequate emotional resources	
Religious conviction	Ignorance and unwillingness to disscuss information within family group
Strong marital relationship prior to onset of MS	Inability or unwillingness to use professional help
Denial of initial stages of the disease ('cushions' shock)	General lack of communication
Steady transition from denial to adjustment and education	
Accurate information enabling realistic expectations	
Avoidance of focusing family life solely around individual with MS (or other neurological deficit)	
Early and continuous professional support	

IMPACT OF NEUROLOGICAL DISEASE AND DISABILITY ON THE FAMILY

Early interventions from specialist nurses, psychologists, occupational therapists, physiotherapists and community health team have been seen as very important in laying the groundwork for the future and in identifying families who may need extra support in their efforts to adapt (MS Forum 1995). An important goal of these interventions is to reinforce positive coping (see Table 11.4). Soderberg (1992) suggests that families also employ two key strategies:

- *Plan for the worst while hoping for the best.* Information about the illness helps family members be more prepared for and less shocked by each symptom or physical change, helps them to make decisions that simplify rather than complicate the future, and enables them to plan financially.
- *Make a place for the neurological condition within the family without giving it more space than it actually needs.* Accommodating the disease enables the needs of other family members

to be met and prevents disruption of the entire family system (Steinglass 1992). In addition, family support needs to take into account the specific needs of other family members.

- *Children.* Although children cope well with a parent's multiple sclerosis, they may report more feelings, fears and coping difficulties than their parents recognise, and they may respond more acutely to mood swings, cognitive impairments or fatigue which can be interpreted by a child as lack of interest or laziness.
- *Spouses.* Couples also have greater success accommodating physical problems than in accommodating mood swings, personality changes and cognitive deficits. This may be compounded if the spouse also has the additional stress of caregiving.
- *Caregivers.* In a comparative study of the physical, social, mental and financial well-being of caregivers, those giving care to people with MS reported similar deficits to those giving care to people with Alzheimer's, reporting deficits in their physical, mental and social well-being plus four times the number of stress symptoms of the general population (Dewis and Niskala 1992).

The professional's role is to enhance a family's understanding of the neurological impairment, how that might affect the person's participation and activity in family life, and identify what support the person and family may need from specialist practitioners, social services and self-help support groups and charities.

QUALITY OF LIFE

Health-related quality of life is recognised as a significant concept in health care, since survival alone may not be the most critical measure. Quality of Life is a descriptive term referring to people's emotional, social and physical well-being, and their ability to function in the ordinary tasks of living (Donald 2000). Health-related quality of life measures explore the impact of a disease and the different treatment options from a perspective of objective functioning and subjective well-being. One of the strengths of a measure is how it enables a carer to monitor and evaluate the effects of a treatment or a condition from the patient's perspective. It generates information important to the multidisciplinary team involved in different aspects of the person's care (Donald 2000). However, boredom often accompanies hospital and nursing home stays and nurses can encourage participation in a range of activities, such as those suggested in Box 11.1, and consult with occupational therapist or family members.

WORK

Work, both paid and unpaid, fulfils a diversity of needs that help increase self-esteem and a sense of being part of a community, a sense of productivity and challenge, and enhances the maintenance of routines and habits. The Disability Discrimination Act 1995 (DDA) was passed to end discrimination that many disabled people faced. It protects disabled people in employment; in their access to goods, facilities and services; in

---

Box 11.1 Everyday leisure activities

Leisure activities
Watching TV/video/cinema
Listening to radio/music
Reading newspapers/magazines/books
Gardening
Baking
Going for a walk
Visiting the pub

Local resources
Local clubs and support groups
Dial-a-Ride service
Travel agencies specialising in holidays for people with disability
Special local facilities

---

the management, buying or renting of land or property; and in education.

Since 1999, the Disability Discrimination Act has required organisations to review access to any of their services, and with the creation of the Disability Rights Commission in 2000, education providers at all levels of education are now required to ensure that they do not discriminate against disabled people. Codes of practice concerning the details of these are available from the Disability Rights Commission.

GARY'S CASE

Gary (see case study in the section on How to Use this Book) is very young and should make a good recovery, but may well have some residual deficits. It may be that in the period of recovery the preoccupation that various professionals have with clinical signs and pathologies, bowels and hygiene, physical tone management and the learning of self-care tasks is not being translated in his mind as the basis from which he can reclaim joy in the quality of his life. It may be helpful to explore with him during the rehabilitation phase possible options for a return to meaningful occupation and taking a realistic view of long-term planning, spending part of the time looking for all examples of skills, interests, abilities and knowledge that can help guide his choices (Cantrell 1997).

DRIVING AND TRANSPORT

Not being able to drive can have a significantly negative effect on a person's mood, motivation and quality of life. Many people with neurological impairment or disease, however, are able to drive again after a medical examination. The Mobility Advice and Vehicle Information Centre (MAVIS) offers people with a disability a full driving ability assessment, will give advice on car adaptations and provide factsheets on applying for a licence and on insurers who offer policies for people with disabilities (Hemihelp 2004).

Seizure and driving

The Driver and Vehicle Licensing Agency (DVLA) requires anyone who has a seizure at any time to stop driving and to inform the Agency. The time off driving will depend on medical investigation and whether seizures have been successfully controlled. The driving licence usually needs to be surrendered for one year. Licences can be reissued if the person has been completely free from seizures for one year, from the date of the last seizure, or has experienced only sleep seizures for three years, and the DVLA is satisfied that the driver is not a source of danger to others. Different types of epilepsy are described in more detail in Chapter 13.

SUMMARY

❏ A range of cognitive and perceptual disturbances affect memory, attention, sequencing, visual perception of depth, figure/ground discrimination, object recognition, spatial orientation and language. Close working with occupational therapy can help retrain these skills.

❏ Neurological impairments are often strongly associated with low or severe depression but it can be difficult to assess for depression because of other motor, perceptual or cognitive deficits. The negative mood can affect recovery, rehabilitation and quality of life, and treatment should be prompt.

❏ Fatigue is common, particularly in multiple sclerosis. Care planning with occupational therapy and activity analysis can help minimise effort needed in daily activities.

❏ Motivation and adaptation can be facilitated by giving information about current care to the patient and family, by referring to support groups and by giving support in finding help and information in overcoming difficulties, for example information about driving and disability and about the Disability Rights Commission.

REFERENCES

Burgess, M. (2002) *Multiple Sclerosis Theory and Practice for Nurses.* Whurr, London.

Cantrell, T. (1997) Work occupation and disability. In Wilson, B. A. and McLellan, D. L. (eds), *Rehabilitation Studies Handbook.* Cambridge University Press, Cambridge, chapter 6.

Dewis, M. E. and Niskala, H. (1992) Nurturing a valuable resource: family caregivers in multiple sclerosis. *Axone* **13**, 87–91.

MS Forum (1995) Impact of multiple sclerosis on the family. In *Psychosocial Factors in Multiple Sclerosis: Proceedings of the MS Forum Modern Management Workshop, Rome*, chapter 5.

Calne, S. M. and Kumar, A. (2003) Nursing care of patients with late stage Parkinson's disease. *Journal of Neuroscience Nursing* **35** (5), 242–51.

Donald, A. (2000) What is quality of life? *Bandolier* **1**, 9, available at www.evidence-based-medicine.co.uk

Edmans, J. *et al.* (2001) *Occupational Therapy and Stroke*. Whurr, London.

Grieve, J. (1993) *Neuropsychology for Occupational Therapists*. Blackwell Science, Oxford.

Griffin, J. and Tyrell, I. (2003) *Human Givens: A New Approach to Emotional Health and Clear Thinking*. Human Givens Publishing, Chalvington.

Hemihelp (2004) *Driving*, Information Sheet, available at www.hemihelp.org.uk

Multiple Sclerosis Society (2001) *Fatigue*, Factsheet. MS Society, London.

Pedretti, L. W. and Early, M. B. (1996) *Occupational Therapy Practice Skills for Physical Dysfunction*. Mosby, St Louis.

RCP (Royal College of Physicians) (1999) *National Clinical Guidelines for Stroke*. RCP, London.

Reed, K. L. (2001) *Quick Reference to Occupational Therapy*. Aspen, Maryland.

Soderberg, J. (1992) MS and the family system. In Kalb, R. C. and Scheinberg, L. (eds), *Multiple Sclerosis and the Family*. Demos, New York.

Steinglass, P. (1992) Multifamily group therapy. In Kalb, R. C. and Scheinberg, L. (eds), *Multiple Sclerosis and the Family*. Demos, New York.

Stuifbergen, A. K. and Rogers, S. (1997) The experience of fatigue and strategies of self care among people with multiple sclerosis. *Applied Nursing Research* **10** (1) 2–10.

Wright, B. and Fletcher, B. L. (1982) Uncovering hidden resources: a challenge in assessment. *Professional Psychology*, **13**, 229.

12 | Expressing Sexuality

INTRODUCTION

Sexuality influences thoughts, feelings, interactions and actions among human beings and motivates people to find love, contact warmth and intimacy in socially and culturally acceptable ways. Concern about altered body image, the physical ability to have sexual intercourse and the self-care abilities needed to present oneself to the world as a sexually attractive being can be problematical aspects of neurological impairment. The resulting loss of confidence can have a debilitating effect on a person's sense of well being and on their personal relationships. A lack of enjoyment in sexual activity can stem from problems with desire, arousal, orgasm and satisfaction originating in psychological distress rather than neurological impairment. At the other end of the scale, a patient may develop strongly disinhibited sexual behaviour following damage to the frontal lobes in the brain through traumatic or acquired brain injury. This also can have a very negative effect on their personal relationships and cause social embarrassment to others. This chapter draws attention to problems commonly experienced by people with neurological impairments.

LEARNING OUTCOMES

❑ Appreciate how neurological impairment can affect a person's physiological and psychological sexuality.

❑ Outline the role of the nurse in helping patients overcome the practical problems of expressing sexuality caused by neurological impairment.

❑ Appreciate the role of counselling skills and behaviour modification in helping patients with hyposexual and hypersexual problems.

PHYSICAL, PSYCHOLOGICAL AND SOCIAL ASPECTS

It has been estimated that over 50% of people with neurological disorders may experience sexual dysfunction, but of these only approximately only 25% express concern about their difficulty. Those who do report a problem may make their own adjustments and not need help (Chandler and Brown 1998). In a study evaluating sexual dysfunction in people with multiple sclerosis, Zorzon *et al.* (2001) found that over 70% had sexual dysfunction and that over time this correlated with bladder function much more strongly than with psychological factors. In a study by Edmans (2001), stroke patients and their partners gave the following reasons as to why their sexual life had deteriorated:

- lack of motivation or interest from either partner;
- physical incapacity of the patient;
- difficulty getting into a comfortable position;
- difficulty getting their partner aroused;
- difficulty due to sensory deficit.

Sexual dysfunction in multiple sclerosis has also been correlated in particular with bowel and bladder symptoms, sensory disturbance of the genitalia, weakness of the pelvic floor and spasticity (Hulter and Lundberg 1995).

LOUISE'S CASE

People with multiple sclerosis report a high degree of sexual dysfunction (Burgess 2002). In the case of Louise (see case study in the section on How to Use this Book), it may be related to primary dysfunction, such as loss of perineal sensation and loss of the ability to experience orgasm, or because of secondary problems such as incontinence, pain or fatigue, and other psychosocial factors such as low self-esteem depression or stress. Improving sexual function relies on improving the contributory factors such as depression or pain, improving the sensation with drug treatment or with vibrators. She could also refer to specific MS websites that deal openly and explicitly with problems of sexual dysfunction, such as the American, Canadian or Australian Multiple Sclerosis Societies websites.

249

ELLA'S CASE

Although Ella (see case study in the section on How to Use this Book) is still in the early days of her stroke recovery, she is very aware of her current loss of continence, the paralysis of part of her body and her communication difficulties. As she recovers, she may have to make significant readjustments, particularly if her husband is going to be involved as her carer in the short or longer term.

FRED'S CASE

Among people with Parkinson's disease, Bronner *et al.* (2004) found that women had most difficulty with arousal, reaching orgasm and low sexual desire. Nearly 70% of the men in the study had erectile dysfunction, with over half reporting sexual dissatisfaction and slightly under half reporting premature ejaculation and/or difficulty reaching orgasm. Bronner *et al.* (2004) also noted that the use of medication and the advanced stage of the disease contributed to dysfunction. This is also true of the anticholinergic medicine such as oxybutinin, which may contribute to erectile dysfunction in men. Fred (see case study in the section on How to Use this Book) may have autonomic dysfunction, depression, fatigue, loss of libido and loss of self-esteem which interferes with his sexual function, there may be difficulties in the relationship, or his wife may also be experiencing fatigue and loss of libido as the caring role takes its toll.

OTHER FACTORS AFFECTING LIBIDO AND SEXUALITY

Physical impairments undoubtedly have an important role in sexual functioning but other aspects are also significant (Abrams 1981; Woollett and Edelmann 1988; Halvorson and Metz 1992; Chandler and Brown 1998). These can include:

- loss of libido associated with depression;
- change in roles within relationship or in the dynamics of relationship;
- whether a marriage began before the onset of disability;
- depression, severe stress states;
- narcotics, sedatives, alcohol, certain antihypertensives, and medications to treat the disease or condition. Antidepressants, particularly serotonin reuptake inhibitors, have been

associated with delayed or absent orgasm, and tricyclic anti-depressants with erectile dysfunction;

- alteration in sexual self-concept includes embarrassment, shame or sense of inadequacy because of body changes such as muscle wasting, spasticity, appliances such as catheters;
- orgasm alterations include problems with ejaculatory function and perception of pleasure associated with orgasm;
- fear and anger from personal conflicts about success and intimacy.

Counselling may be helpful for psychological or relationship difficulties as well as for treating the depression that may further compromise sexual activity. Evidence to support effective interactions with women who experience loss of libido or difficulty achieving orgasm is lacking. For vaginal dryness and pain during intercourse, water-based lubricants may help (Burgess 2000).

ERECTILE DYSFUNCTION

Physiologically the reflex centres for sexual function reside in the lower thoracic, lumbar and sacral spine. Damage to the neurones in this region can cause erectile dysfunction although the desire may be present. For men with erectile dysfunction there are a number of options (MST 2000):

- intracaverosal alprostadil;
- intraurethral applications;
- vacuum constrictor devices;
- penile prosthesis implants;
- oral medications such as Viagra, which can give improvement in penetration and maintenance of erections.

MARK AND GARY'S CASES

Both Mark and Gary (see case studies in the section on How to Use this Book) will need support in regaining sexual confidence as their rehabilitation progresses, most probably requiring a combination of approaches, including identification of any physical or neurological cause, and whether this can be improved by treatment, whether drug treatments are causing loss of libido, and whether the men see counselling as a helpful option.

MENSTRUATION, CONTRACEPTION AND PREGNANCY

Research is limited on the complex area of reproduction and neurological disease, and patients should always have access to specialist help. The research that has been done, however, shows that multiple sclerosis is more common in women and that they often experience worsening of their symptoms just before menstruation. Contraceptive choices should always be discussed with a physician, bearing in mind that drugs such as antibiotics, phenytoin and carbamezepine may reduce contraceptive effectiveness. During pregnancy itself, women who have multiple sclerosis are much less likely to suffer a relapse, and although the risk increases slightly in the three months after delivery, this soon settles (Vukusic *et al.* 2004). For women who have epilepsy, the pregnancy, medication and seizure control need to be monitored carefully.

ROLE OF THE NURSE

The topic of sexuality can be a difficult one to broach for either patient or nurse. Burgess (2000) suggests that sexual function should be addressed in the same matter-of-fact way as bowel function and bladder function are discussed, and that even if the individual nurse feels insufficiently skilled to offer help in this area, they should be aware of to whom the patient should be referred for appropriate advice (for example, consultant neurologist, urologist, nurse specialist, self-help group). The P-LI-SS-IT model – (Anon 1976) can be used to explore different levels of intervention for different levels of expertise, as shown in Box 12.1.

INTERVENTIONS

In general settings, nurses can help people to begin to resolve some of the difficulties they may be having in expressing their sexuality by:

- noticing clues about how the person is feeling about themselves or their partners;
- acknowledging a person's concern and developing a listening attitude to help people feel more confident about voicing their concerns;

- when appropriate and if the patient wishes, providing information about areas of concern and making referrals to support groups. For example, if someone has an indwelling catheter they may not realise that it is possible to have sexual intercourse with the drainage tube removed and the catheter tube secured with a spigot;
- providing holistic care that addresses activities that influence how someone feels about themselves, such as assisting them with washing, dressing and grooming that enables the person to have as much autonomy as possible in their presentation of self;
- providing specific suggestions about how to manage continence problems, fatigue, positioning to avoid spasm and pain;
- referring the patient and partner for specialised help, such as psychosexual therapy, if they wish.

DISINHIBITION AND HYPERSEXUALITY

Hypersexuality can be associated with dementia, brain injury, stroke and Parkinson's disease. It occurs because of combined loss of inhibitions and memory impairments. The normal pattern of sexual behaviour may be altered with diseases of the limbic system. Any condition affecting the frontal lobes may disinhibit, with indiscriminate sexuality. Temporal lobe epilepsy can also be associated with hypersexuality. Some people with neurotrauma may be vulnerable because of the loss of complex reasoning skills and the loss of social inhibition, and people may take advantage of them financially, socially or sexually.

Disinhibited behaviours may include:

- using sexual slang and oaths;
- masturbating in public areas;
- requesting sexual favours;
- making lewd comments;
- inappropriately touching breasts and buttocks (now considered sexual harassment at work (Libbus and Bowman 1994).

These behaviours can be very difficult to deal with. The nurse's relationship with a patient affords access to areas of a patient's

---

Box 12.1 The P-LI-SS-IT model

Level 1 Permission (P)
Using basic counselling skills of open-ended questioning and reflection to create a comfortable safe environment, so that the patient understands that it is acceptable for them to discuss any sexual problems if they wish. At this level a nurse may simply acknowledge that problems are common and be able to provide information leaflets and put the person in touch with people or organisations that can offer further help.

Level 2 Limited Information (LI)
A nurse working at this level will have sufficient knowledge of the problem, such as erectile dysfunction, to be able to discuss some options.

Level 3 Specific Suggestions (SS)
A nurse working at this level will probably be a specialist in the field, such MS Nurse Specialist, Parkinson's Disease Nurse Specialist, and have a wide knowledge base and experience upon which to draw and be able to offer specific suggestions in relation to the problem.

Level 4 Intensive Therapy (IT)
A nurse working at this level will have had specific training in counselling and helping people with complex interpersonal relationships and psychological aspects of sexual function.

---

body that are normally very private, and people with a cognitive disturbance of disinhibition may misconstrue essential nursing activities such as catheter care or continence management.

Managing disinhibition and hypersexuality
The level of the disturbance will indicate whether specialist help is needed, and in many cases the behaviour can be modified using behavioural techniques. These include the following:

- Withdrawing positive reinforcement, such as attention, and being aware that during apparently informal interactions with patients, a nurse's response, even if angry, may reinforce behaviours for better or worse.
- If touched inappropriately, tell the patient that it is inappropriate and withdraw if the behaviour persists. 'I am your nurse and it not appropriate for you to touch me in that way.'
- During activities such as washing and dressing, place a washcloth or item of clothing in the patient's hands and encourage them to wash and dress themself.
- Ensure that behaviour modification is included in the care plan and that the team adopts a consistent approach.

HARRY'S CASE

It is important that Harry's care plan gives specific guidance on how to respond to his sexually inappropriate behaviour (see case study in the section on How to Use this Book) so that all nurses are consistent in their approach. It is most effective if nurses remain calm but firm, and by facial expression, tone of voice and words deliver the judgement that the behaviour is not appropriate. They take the opportunity to reorientate, explaining that he has had a brain injury and that he is recovering but it is not appropriate that he touches the nurses in that way. If Harry's behaviour does not improve he will need to be assessed by a clinical psychologist to explore other behaviour modification techniques that nurses can use.

SUMMARY

❏ Sexuality can be disrupted by physiological impairment to functioning of the nervous system or by psychological disturbances and loss of confidence about attractiveness.
❏ Nurses can help in resolving practical problems such as bowel and bladder management, managing fatigue, spasticity and pain.
❏ Counselling skills in listening and responding and using behaviour modification strategies can help nurses manage patients with erectile dysfunction, loss of libido and confidence in sexual activity, disinhibition and hypersexuality.

REFERENCES

Abrams, K. S. (1981) The impact on marriages of adult onset paraplegia. *Paraplegia* **19** (4), 253–9.

Anon (1976) The P-LI-SS-IT model: a proposed conceptual scheme for behavioural treatment of sexual problems. *Journal of Sex Education Therapy* **2**, 1–15.

Bronner, G., Royter, V., Koryczyn, A. and Giladi, N. (2004) Sexual dysfunction in Parkinson's disease. *Journal of Sex and Marital Therapy* **30** (2), 95–105.

Burgess, M. (2000) *Multiple Sclerosis Theory and Practice for Nurses.* Whurr, London.

Chandler, B. J. and Brown, S. (1998) Sex and relationship dysfunction in neurological disability. *Journal of Neurological Neurosurgical Psychiatry* **65** (6), 877–80.

Edmans, J. (2001) *Occupational Therapy and Stroke.* Whurr, London.

Halvorson, J. G. and Metz, M. E. (1992) Sexual dysfunction. Part 1: Classification, aetiology and pathogenesis. *Journal of the American Board of Family Practitioners* **5** (1), 51–61.

Hulter, B. M. and Lundberg, P. O. (1995) Sexual dysfunction in women with advanced multiple sclerosis. *Journal of Neurological Psychiatry* **59** (1), 83–6.

Libbus, M. K. and Bowman, K. G. (1994) Sexual harassment of female registered nurses in hospitals. *Journal of Nursing Administration* **24** (6), 26–31.

MST (Multiple Sclerosis Trust) (2000) *Multiple Sclerosis Information for Health and Social Care Professionals.* Multiple Sclerosis Trust, Letchworth.

Vukusic, S., Hutchinson, M., Hours, M., Moreau, T., Cortinovis-Tourniaire, P., Adeleine, P., Confavreux, C. and the Pregnancy in Multiple Sclerosis Group (2004) Pregnancy and multiple sclerosis (the PRIMS study): clinical predictors of post-partum relapse. *Brain* **127** (6), 1353–60.

Woollett, S. L. and Edelmann, R. J. (1988) Marital satisfaction in individuals with multiple sclerosis and their partners: its interactive effect with life satisfaction, social networks and disability. *Sex Marital Therapy* **3** (2), 191–6.

Zorzon, M., Zivadinov, R., Monti Bragadani, L., De Masi, R., Nasuelli, D. and Cazzato, G. (2001) Sexual dysfunction in multiple sclerosis: a two-year follow-up study. *Journal of Neurological Science* **187** (1/2), 1–5.

Sleeping

13

INTRODUCTION

Sleeping is the naturally restorative activity of body and mind that is usually related to the 24-hour light–dark cycle. Sleep enhances tissue growth and restoration, and protein synthesis is increased while cell work is decreased. The rhythmical nature of the sleep–wake cycle is influenced by neurochemical, physiological, psychological, developmental and temporal factors, and most people fall in the 6–8 hours night range. Although the mechanism of the sleep–wake cycle is not well understood, it can be disrupted in neurological disease not only from discomforts but also from damage to the brain that disrupts the biological clock, interferes with the perception of night and day, and causes agitation and psychological distress. Because nurses are often present in the care setting over twenty-four hours, seven days a week, they are in a good position to assess whether patients have a disordered sleep pattern that may be exacerbating other discomforts.

This chapter focuses on the normal sleep cycle, the factors that can disrupt it, the effects of disturbed sleep and the nursing measures that may alleviate the discomforts and help restore pattern. In addition, this chapter outlines seizure activity as a possible source of temporary altered consciousness.

LEARNING OUTCOMES

❏ Understand the importance of sleep cycles and patterns in physical and psychological well-being.
❏ Describe the external and internal sources of sleep disturbance and the three main classifications of sleep disturbance.
❏ Appreciate states of temporarily altered consciousness related to seizure activity.

❏ Outline pharmacological and non-pharmacological interventions to help promote sleep.

STAGES AND STATES OF SLEEP

The neural control of the sleep–wake cycle is thought to lie in the anterior hypothalamus (Adams and Victor 1994). There are two types of sleep: rapid eye movement (REM) sleep, also known as dreaming sleep, and non-rapid eye movement (NREM) sleep, also known as slow wave sleep (SWS) and from which it is difficult to rouse people. During a night's sleep a person will cycle through these stages, and the proportions of REM to NREM periods and the total length of sleep vary according to age, individuality, and psychological and physical well-being. It is thought that the stages of NREM sleep correlate with body restoration, based on the physiological, endocrine and EEG changes. The REM state is thought to function as a way restoring peace of mind (Griffin 1997), and that in depressed people much of the feeling of fatigue and exhaustion after a night's sleep is caused by excessive amounts of REM sleep. The role of dreams in well-being is widely researched and is a subject surrounded by different beliefs that people hold about the dreams' significance. However, it is known that night sedation can alter the characteristics of sleep since it interferes with neurochemical regulation and may undermine the function of dream sleep (Griffin 1997).

Because REM sleep is accompanied by a paralysis of the anti-gravity muscles, if someone wakes up before coming out of REM sleep they may be badly frightened. This can be part of normal experience, but can be additionally terrifying for people with existing motor problems.

Disturbances of sleep pattern

Sleep disturbance is classified in three groups:

- disorders of excessive somnolence (DOES);
- disorders of initiation and maintenance of sleep (DIMS) such as insomnia;
- abnormal behaviours caused by the sleep disorders such as sleepwalking or night terrors.

Excessive somnolence (DOES) includes falling asleep during activities such as eating or driving as well as sleeping during the day while at rest. It often follows stroke and traumatic brain injury in the early days (Masel *et al.* 2001), but can also be caused by antidepressants, muscle relaxants, anti-Parkinsonian drugs (Thorpy 2004) and sedatives; it may also be indicative of depression. Sleep apnoea, caused by partial obstruction of the airway, may also follow stroke. Fred (see case study in the section on How to Use this Book) may well have a very disturbed sleep–wake cycle, as his anti-Parkinson medication may be causing drowsiness during the day, but causing hallucinations and vivid dreams during the night.

Someone with *insomnia (DIMS)* finds it difficult to fall asleep, has difficulty staying asleep and/or wakes up early. Insomnia often has a psychological component.

A person with *parasomnia* may experience sleepwalking, body jerks and startles while asleep, nightmares and night terrors.

Most disturbances will fall into one or more of the above three categories and it is important to make good observations and thorough assessment, and to plan interventions based on an understanding of the problem underlying the disturbed pattern. It will usually be found that a combination of both intrinsic and extrinsic factors are responsible for a disturbance in sleep pattern (Rogers 2001). Such factors include:

- physiological discomforts, for example pain, nocturia;
- emotional and psychological disturbance, for example worry, acute anxiety, stress;
- effects of neurological impairments such as dementia, Parkinson's disease, brain injury, sleep-related epilepsy;
- arousal disorders causing sleepwalking and nightmares;
- problems with sleep–wake transitions, including sleep talking, nocturnal leg cramps, and startles;
- the circle of lost sleep pattern and how its ill-effects maintain the vicious circle.

Effects of sleep deprivation

The effects of sleep deprivation exacerbate existing neurological problems and include:

- irritability;
- fatigue;
- inability to concentrate;
- disorientation;
- reduced performance of mental and physical tasks;
- occasionally illusions, delusions or paranoid thoughts.

In addition, the deprivation of REM sleep can increase anxiety, and lead to overeating and hypersexuality, while excessive dream sleep can be associated with depression (Griffin 1997).

People with ongoing neurological disease or long-term neurological impairment have been found to suffer proportions of sleep disorders and disturbance that were sufficiently severe to interfere with recovery and well-being rehabilitation (Drake and Bradshaw 1999; Fichtenberg *et al.* 2002).

SEIZURES
A seizure is an abnormal and excessive discharge of neuronal activity that results in an altered state of brain function and, usually, awareness.

Epilepsy
Epilepsy is a chronic tendency to seizure as a repetitive occurrence. The manifestation of seizure depends on which neurones are involved and how far and how quickly the discharge spreads or extends (Shorvon and Walker 1999). Although no specific cause can be found for epilepsy, in most cases the major risk factors for neurological patients' developing seizures include:

- traumatic brain injury;
- infections of the central nervous system such as meningitis, abscess;
- primary and metastic brain tumours;
- cerebro-vascular disease such as stroke or haemorrhage.

Seizures are classified in different ways, and close observation, documentation of seizure activity can help classify the nature of the seizure, and its appropriate treatment. An example of such an observation chart is shown in Fig 13.1. If nurses

Seizure Activity Chart

SEIZURE ACTIVITY CHART

Patient name: _____ Ward: _____ Patient Hospital Number: _____

* Please tick appropriate box

			Date:								
			Time:								
			Duration:								
PRE-ICTAL	(specify)	Unusual behaviour, e.g. mood change, fear									
	(specify)	Part of body where seizure began; head, limbs, uni/bilateral									
ICTAL	SENSORY*	Pins & needles									
		Numbness									
		Smell									
		Taste									
	VISUAL*	Bright flashes									
		Hallucinations									
	EYE MOVEMENTS*	Fluttering									
		Rolling									
		Staring									
		Closed									
		Turns to side									
	PUPIL RESPONSE*	Size									
		Reaction									
	BREATHING*	Irregular									
		Laboured									
		Rapid/slow									
		Noisy									
		Cyanosis									
		Sats (%)									
	VOCALISATION*	None									
		Cry let out									
		Mumbles									
		Grunts									
		Repeats phrases									
	MOTOR*	Loss of tone / fall									
		Twitching									
		Rigidity									
		Jerking									
	INVOLUNTARY MOTOR*	Lip smacking									
		Chewing									
		Fumble / plucks									
		Grimacing									
	LEVEL OF CONSCIOUSNESS*	Responsive									
		Unresponsive									
		Confused									
		Dreamstate									
	OTHER*	Dizzy									
		Sweating									
		Tachycardia									
		Excessive saliva									
		Tongue-biting									
		Incontinent faeces									
		Incontinent urine									
		Bizarre behaviour									
POST-ICTAL	*	Sleeping									
		Amnesic									
		Headache									
		Nausea									
		Weakness/ Muscle ache									
		Confused									

Salford Royal Hospitals NHS
NHS Trust

Figure 13.1 Seizure activity chart (reproduced with permission from Salford Royal Hospitals Trust).

PHASES OF SEIZURE ACTIVITY

PRODOMAL	Involves mood or behaviour changes that may precede seizure by several hours / days.
PRE-ICTAL/ AURA	Premonition of impending seizure activity, may be visual, auditory, gustatory or olfactory – refers to symptoms immdiately before possible loss of consciousness and will localise the attack to its point of origin in the nervous system.
ICTAL	The seizure activity.
POST-ICTAL	A period of possible confusion / irritability that occurs after the seizure.

CLASSIFICATION OF SEIZURES

PARTIAL

SIMPLE PARTIAL: involves part of brain, consciousness not impaired. Often divided into temporal, frontal, parietal and occipital lobe seizures depending where seizure starts.

COMPLEX PARTIAL: consciousness is impaired. Common for automatisms to occur i.e. behaviours appear purposeful but may be bizarre e.g. fumbling, speaking nonsense, undressing.

N.B. SECONDARY GENERALISED: can result from a simple or complex partial seizure. Results from the spread of the seizure throughout both halves of the brain.

GENERALISED

ABSENCE: (petit-mal) short blank spells.

MYOCLONIC: brief jerks of whole limb or whole of body.

CLONIC: intermittent muscular contraction and relaxation (jerking).

TONIC: continuous muscular contractions (stiffening).

TONIC-CLONIC: (grand-mal) body stiffens and jerks uncontrollably.

ATONIC: (drop attack) loss of muscle tone, falls to ground and able to get up again almost immediately.

Seizure Activity Chart

Figure 13.1 *Continued*

suspect that patients are experiencing temporary disturbances of consciousness that could be seizure activity, even while patients are asleep, that possibility should be investigated.

- *Generalised seizure* is the term used to describe discharges that occur simultaneously throughout the cortex and consciousness is impaired.
- *Absences* are where there are blank spells that may or may not be accompanied by abnormal muscle tone, or automatic activities such as fumbling or swallowing or chewing.
- *Tonic–clonic seizures* are where the patient, falls and goes stiff, followed by rhythmic movements of arms and legs, grunting, foaming at the mouth, incontinence and tongue biting. As the patient recovers, there may deep respiration, confusion, headache and a need to sleep.
- *Partial seizures* begin in a specific group of neurones and may then spread.
- In *simple partial seizures*, consciousness may not be impaired there may be focal motor signs, autonomic signs such as flushing, pallor, sweating or psychic symptoms such as deja vue, illusions or hallucinations
- In *complex partial seizures*, consciousness may be impaired and there may be automatic activity such as chewing, swallowing, plucking or fumbling with clothes.

Epilepsy Action (2003) gives the following first aid guidance for tonic–clonic seizure activity:

Do
- Stay calm.
- Loosen any tight clothing around the neck.
- Protect from injury.
- Cushion the head if on the ground.
- Place in the recovery position when convulsive movements subside.
- Protect airway, stay with person and act as a witness of the seizure.

Don't
- Try to restrain the person.
- Put anything in the mouth or between the teeth.

- Move the person unless in danger.
- Give anything to drink until fully recovered.

Occasionally the management of seizure activity becomes uncontrolled, often because of concurrent illness, changes in drug therapy or some other underlying problem and may develop into a medical emergency, status epilepticus. This is associated with significant mortality and morbidity if not treated properly (NICE 2004). Control of status epilepticus needs intravenous access and specialised clinical care. However, first aid treatment outside a suitable care setting can include the administration rectal diazepam of 10–20 mg.

If the seizure activity is partial it is still important to observe and record the circumstances and manifestations as this can help in developing seizure control. In addition, people who suffer sleep-related seizure activity may have improvements in their quality of life if this nocturnal activity is recognised and treated.

Vegetative state

Vegetative state is a sustained alteration in the level of con-sciousness described as a state of complete unawareness of the self and the environment, accompanied by sleep–wake cycles, with either complete or partial preservation of hypothalamic and brain stem autonomic functions. When it lasts for more than one month it is called *persistent vegetative state* (Hickey 1997). Life expectancy is much reduced, with survival unusual beyond ten years. See Boxes 13.1 and 13.2.

Locked-in syndrome

Locked-in syndrome is a condition of severe paralysis of motor neurones that makes voluntary movement and communication impossible. Consciousness and cognition are intact, as is breath-ing. Damage to motor pathways occurs because of interruption at the level of the pons, motor neurone disease, neuromuscular-blocking drugs, some cases of cerebrovascular disease, poliomyelitis or myasthenia gravis.

Box 13.1 Criteria for persistent vegetative state

- Shows no evidence of sustained, reproducible, purposeful or voluntary behavioural responses to visual, auditory, tactile or noxious stimuli.
- Shows no evidence of language comprehension or expression.
- Shows no bowel or bladder control.
- Demonstrates variable patterns of preserved cranial nerve and spinal reflexes and primitive reflexes such as sucking.
- Maintains vital signs and spontaneous respirations.
- Has eyes open and spontaneous eye movement. Sometimes the patient's eyes appear to follow people in the room but the patient is unable to follow a command or look in a particular direction.

Box 13.2 Causes and outcome of persistent vegetative state

• Acute traumatic and non-traumatic brain injury	Recovery unlikely after 12 months
• Degenerative and metabolic brain disorders	Recovery unlikely after 3 months
• Severe congenital malformation of the nervous system	Recovery rare after several months

---

Low awareness states

Low awareness states are less rigidly defined and can be used for a range of low awareness levels that patients have following injury as it can be very difficult to feel sure about how much sensory, verbal, perceptual and cognitive activity the person experiences. Some patients may have a drowsy form and appear to spend much of their time dozing. Others may have a profound motor restlessness that takes no account of clock and can pace ceaselessly or call out loudly at any time of the day or night and show very little awareness of their surroundings. In either case, it is important to try to build into the routine a sense of night and day, to protect the patient from exhaustion and from deteriorating further. For example, it may be difficult to assess whether Anwah (see case study in the section on How to Use this Book) experiences night and day, but effort should be made to ensure that structure and stimulation give her as strong as possible a sense of day, and that night-time is conveyed by low light, quietness and perhaps a sleep system as in Figure 13.2. This can help support her in a therapeutic position and will confer a sense of boundary and security. Pillows can also be used if a custom-built system is not available.

NURSING ASSESSMENT

Nursing assessment needs to include both subjective reports and, as far as possible, observation. Frost (1998) posits that subjective reports of sleep are often incorrect, but this is actually difficult to be sure about, and an observer's report that a person

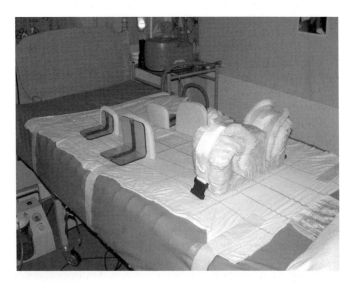

Figure 13.2 Sleep support system (reproduced with permission from Priory Healthcare).

has slept well may be just as incorrect. Even so, many people who feel they have insomnia are shown in sleep laboratories to have normal sleep. Neurological patients with excessive sleepiness may be unaware that they fall asleep at inappropriate times, and people with sleep apnoea may be unaware of the sleep disturbance it causes. A good sleep assessment should include both self-report and observations covering the following:

- What time the person usually goes to bed, whether they waken in the night and what time they waken in the morning.
- Do they take any medications or drinks that contain caffeine or alcohol before bed?
- Do they toss and turn? Are there periodic leg movement or jerking movements?
- Are their periods of loud snoring or long pauses between breaths?
- Have all the recommended practices for position, posture and support been implemented?
- Do they have any bladder or bowel discomforts?
- Is the pain relief effective?
- What medications are they on and might these cause excessive sleep, disturbed sleep or interference with dream sleep?
- Do they have psychological needs that are not being met?
- Is the sleep pattern poor enough to make them feel sleep deprived and exacerbate the neurological impairment?
- Is there a physical or social environmental factor that they are finding disturbing?
- Does the setting have adequate resources of pillows, supporting devices, blankets, nightlights and noise-reducing measures?

INTERVENTIONS

Interventions are individualised to patient need and many patients may have come to accept a measure of sleep disturbance as an inevitable consequence of their condition. In many cases, the 'expert patient' is able to guide nurses in measures that help, such as position routine, meeting elimination needs during the night and alleviating other factors that may be interfering with sleep. For less participative patients the nurse may need to try a few different approaches before a better pattern is established. In addition to making provision to meet basic comfort, nutritional needs, access to toilet or commode during the night and other sensible sleep-promoting measures, nursing management might include specifically:

- *Sleep apnoea* – careful head positioning at night; sometimes positive airway pressure at night, occasionally respiratory stimulants depending on severity.
- *Insomnia* – modifications to routine such as bathing before bed, relaxation techniques, counselling if the patient wants it, short-term use of night-time sedation.
- *Parasomnias and nocturnal seizures* – recognition and treatment of the underlying factors that may be causing disturbance, such as medication, emotional or psychological distress.

FRED'S CASE

Fred is clearly distressed at night and it may take a few weeks to clear his hallucinating, while the loss of his motor ability is almost immediate, and he may become even more frightened by his increasing dependence. Nurses need to maintain a calm and reassuring presence and to offer whatever help they can. This may include finding the time to listen to him and to his fears, keeping a light on to reduce shadows that may be misinterpreted. He could take the last dose of levodopa several hours before bedtime, and ensure that he is not hungry before going to bed. Watching television in bed may overstimulate his visual imagination. Night sedation and any antipsychotic medication should be given to him promptly. A suitable bed, such as a profiling bed, enables position change, and low-resistance nightwear, such as satin pyjamas, reduces resistance as he changes position. In addition, the daytime drowsiness could be managed by providing a structure to the day that allows time to carry out his activities, with reasonable rest periods but with enough stimulation to ensure that boredom does not exacerbate his drowsiness. This may be difficult to achieve on general wards, but nursing staff could ensure that he has free time during which family and visitors could help him keep occupied and stimulated.

HARRY'S CASE

Harry (see case study in the section on How to Use this Book) is showing a very disturbed sleep pattern. The fact that he is noisy and wandering at night may have a number of contributory factors. He could be having frightening flashbacks and thoughts. He could also be persevarating (repetitive utterances or actions). He may, for example, be shouting 'help me help me help me' and continue saying this even when the nurse begins to try to help him. With impaired processing and agitation he will rely on instinct to interact with others and closely mirror the attitude and mood of the person he is interacting with. It is important, therefore, that the nurse conveys patience and care, rather than walks in with arms folded and saying in loud voice, 'Now what's all this noise about?' Such action will distress him and send him the message 'I am angry', and he may mirror that mood and become angry as well as agitated. It is important to orientate him, tell him who and where he is, that he is safe and ask if there is anything you can do to help him. If the sleep pattern is lost completely and he is burning up calories restlessly during the day, he may need very short term drug treatment, such as zopiclone which is non-addictive and has a minimal hangover effect. In addition, discuss with him and his family his usual sleeping pattern and try to re-establish this by structuring his twenty-four hours. Also, try as far as possible to ensure the environment gives 'night-time' signals such as curtains closed, no noisy talking, low lighting. If the pattern changes and he begins sleeping very heavily at night, the concern about a brain-injured patient is that he may be having seizure activity during the night or he may be going to bed having had a seizure (post-ictal) that has been missed. Another possibility is that he may have been prescribed anticonvulsants that are making him very drowsy. To monitor this, nurses should check to see whether he has been incontinent during the night, observe his behaviour in the evening before he goes to bed for signs of seizure activity and see if there is any correlation between this symptom and when anticonvulsant medication was changed or prescribed. A further possibility may be that overactivity is causing excessive exhaustion in relation to his energy reserves and nutritional intake.

SUMMARY

❏ Sleep cycles consist of alternating periods of NREM and REM sleep, during which protein increase assists tissue regeneration and dream sleep restores mental clarity.

❏ External environments disturb sleep, internal sources include psychological discomfort or distress, neuronal damage disturbing sense of clock or physiological discomforts from nocturia or pain.

❏ The three main classifications of sleep disturbance are: excessive sleepiness (DOES), insomnia (DIMS) and parasomnias, such as sleepwalking.

❏ Seizure activity can occur at any time of the day or night; it needs to be observed and recorded carefully to help manage and control the seizure activity.

❏ Interventions need to ensure that there are sufficient resources to allow correct positioning and comfort at night, and that account is taken of the side effects of some of the drugs prescribed to manage the condition.

REFERENCES

Adams, R. D. and Victor, M. (1994) *Principles of Neurology Companion Handbook*, 5th edn. McGraw-Hill, New York.

Drake, A. and Bradshaw, D. (1999) Sleep disturbances following traumatic brain injury. *Brain Injury Source*, no. 3. Brain Injury Association, Alexander.

Epilepsy Action (2003) *Epilepsy: A Teachers Guide*, available at http://www.epilepsy.org.uk

Fichtenberg, N. L., Zafonte, R. D., Putnam, S., Mann, N. R. and Millard, A. E. (2002) Sleep apnoea and sleep–wake disturbances in stroke patients. *Brain Injury* **16** (3), 197–206.

Frost, J. D. (1998) Sleep disorders. In Rolak, L. A. (ed.) *Neurology Secrets*, 2nd edn. Hanley & Belfus, Philadelphia, chapter 22.

Griffin, J. (1997) *The Origin of Dreams*. The Therapist Ltd, Chalvington.

Hickey, J. V. (1997) *The Clinical Practice of Neurological and Neurosurgical Nursing*, 4th edn. Lippincott, Philadelphia.

Masel, B. E., Scheibel, R. S., Kimbark, T. and Kuna, S. T. (2001) Excessive daytime sleepiness in adults with brain injury. *Archives of Physical Medicine and Rehabilitation* **82** (11), 1526–32.

NICE (2004) *The Epilepsies: The Diagnosis and Management of the Epilepsies in Adults and Children in Primary and Secondary Care*, NICE Guideline. National Institute for Clinical Excellence, London, available at http://www.nice.org.uk

Rogers, A. E. (2001) Rhythmic alterations in loss of consciousness. In Stewart-Amidei, C. and Kunkel, J. A. (eds) *AANN's Neuroscience Nursing*, 2nd edn. W. B. Saunders, New York, chapter 9.

Shorvon, S. and Walker, M. (1999) *MIMS Guide to Epilepsy*. Glaxo Wellcome, Uxbridge.

Thorpy, M. J. (2004) Sleep disorders in Parkinson's disease. *Clinical Cornerstone* **6** (Supplement 1A), S7–S15.

14 | Dying

INTRODUCTION

For many neurological patients there is no cure for the disease or no way of reversing the damage to the nerves caused by degeneration, infection inflammation, or injury to nerve structures. In these circumstances, the goal of palliative care is to achieve the best quality of life for patients and their families. Progressive neurological disease such as motor neurone disease, Parkinson's disease or progressive multiple sclerosis can render a person entirely dependent on ventilatory and nutritional support, and the ethical dilemmas that these interventions may bring. Other neurological diseases or conditions can make people more vulnerable to chest infection, pneumonia and other indirect cause of death.

The process of dying inevitably leads an individual to greater levels of dependence on others, not only for physical care but also for emotion and spiritual support. Individuals have different needs in this respect when living through the process of dying, which may take days, weeks, months or years once an illness is classed as terminal. The symptomatic relief is known as palliative care; it concentrates on the quality of life and alleviation of distressing symptoms for people with a progressive and incurable disorder. Terminal care addresses difficult legal and ethical situations about withholding and withdrawing life-prolonging treatments, advance directives, refusal of treatment, physician-assisted suicide and euthanasia. Many neurological patients and their families will have lived with their disease for a long time before the dying process ensues and may have given some thought to these issues.

The focus of this chapter is on the emotional and physical support that neurological patients may need in palliative care and the two main end-of-life issues of withdrawal of ventilatory support and withdrawal of enteral feeding. While it is beyond the scope of a small book such as this to explore these issues in any depth, the role of the nurse is outlined, but this will need to be supplemented with wider reading of the ethical and legal issues mentioned. The definitions of the terms as used in this chapter are made clearer in Box 14.1.

LEANING OUTCOMES
❏ Appreciate the role of the nurse in the palliative care of people with progressive neurological disease.
❏ Discuss aspects of grief and grieving and the role of the nurse.
❏ Raise awareness of aspects of informed consent, capacity to consent, refusal of treatment, living wills and advance directives concerning ventilatory and nutritional support via a tube.

PALLIATIVE CARE AND TERMINAL CARE
The neurological conditions which give rise to ethical/legal and palliative care issues include persistent vegetative state, motor neurone disease, advanced Parkinson's disease and brain tumours, although other neurological impairments may eventually lead to the need for palliative care, as shown in Table 14.1. The settings in which people are nursed vary greatly, but a survey carried out by a collaborative forum of neurological charities has shown that there is a general lack of awareness of the needs of people with dementia and other neurological conditions in general hospitals, primary care settings, nursing homes and hospices (Neurological Alliance 2001a,b). Suffering in a terminally ill patient derives from physical distress and unmet psychological needs (Chapman and Gavrin 1995) which can be very complex in advanced neurological disease (see Table 14.1). The main problems for this group are the low number of specialist units and services and the difficulty of accessing them. While these units may be accessed relatively easily by a patient with a rarer neurological disease, access is less easy for those with the more common conditions of dementia, stroke epilepsy, Parkinson's disease, brain injury and multiple sclerosis. In addition, the development of an acute complication such as pneumonia may mean the patient is

Box 14.1 Definitions (BMA n.d.)

Terminal illness

A terminal illness is inevitably progressive, resulting in death. Treatment may alleviate symptoms or slow progression of the illness but cannot provide a cure. Some supporters of euthanasia or assisted suicide specify that only terminally ill people, or only people with a terminal illness who are expected to die within a specified time period, should be considered eligible if such procedures were legalised.

Palliative care

The active total care of patients whose disease is not responsive to curative treatment. Control of pain, or other symptoms, and of psychological, social and spiritual problems, is paramount. The goal of palliative care is achievement of the best quality of life for patients and their families (World Health Organization definition).

Advance statements

An expression of views, by competent individuals, concerning treatment options likely to arise later when their decision-making capacity has been lost. Advance directives, or refusals, are a subset of advance statements, in which treatments are refused in advance. Competently made advance directives, applicable to the circumstances, are legally binding upon clinicians.

Non-treatment

(a) Refusal of treatment

Competent adults have the right to refuse any treatment, including life-prolonging procedures. The BMA does not consider valid treatment refusal by a patient to be suicide. Respecting a competent, informed patient's treatment refusal is not assisting suicide.

(b) Withdrawing/withholding life-prolonging medical treatment

Not all treatment with the potential to prolong life has to be provided in all circumstances, especially if its effect is seen as extending the dying process. Cardiopulmonary resuscitation of a terminally ill cancer patient is an extreme example. In deciding which treatment should be offered, the expectation must be that the advantages outweigh the drawbacks for the individual patient.

Double effect
The principle of double effect provides the justification for the provision of medical treatment which has bad effects where the intention is to provide an overall good effect. The principle permits an act which foreseeably has both good and bad effects provided that the good effect is the reason for acting (and is not caused by the bad). A common example is the provision of essential pain relieving drugs in terminal care at the risk of shortening life.

Euthanasia
Euthanasia is a deliberate act or omission whose primary intention is to end another's life. Literally, it only means a gentle or easy death but has come to signify a deliberate intervention with the intention to kill someone, often described as the 'mercy killing' of people in pain with terminal illness. Discussion is complicated by the qualifiers 'voluntary', 'involuntary' and 'non-voluntary' used to indicate the degree of patient involvement. Many advocates of euthanasia limit their support to the 'voluntary' category, where death is brought about at the patient's request. 'Non-voluntary euthanasia' is used to describe the killing of a patient who does not have the capacity to request or consent to it, including, for example, babies. 'Involuntary euthanasia' describes when competent people are killed against their will or without their consent. All categories are legally prohibited. 'Active' and 'passive' are also often applied to describe the extent of the doctor's role. Like many other bodies, including the House of Lords Select Committee on Medical Ethics, the BMA has long taken the view that such terms are ambiguous and unhelpful. Confusion may also arise when the withdrawing or withholding of life-prolonging treatment which is not providing a benefit to the patient is described as 'passive euthanasia'.

Table 14.1 Common problems in advanced and terminal neurological conditions.

Problems	Related potential problems and quality of life	Palliation and treatment	Ethical issues
Spasticity	Pain, reduced mobility, activity and function	Antispasticity medication. Analgesia. Physiotherapy	Informed consent
Dysphagia	Malnutrition, risk for aspiration pneumonia, poor mouth hygiene, dental caries, dry and cracked lips	Gastrostomy feeding, jejunostomy feeding. Nutritional assessment and evaluation, mouth care	Withholding, initiating and withdrawing treatment. Advance directives. Informed consent
Dysarthria and aphasia	Frustration, depression, loss of confidence, relationship with family and friends	Pictorial and other non-verbal communication. Skilled assessment and intervention by speech and language therapist. Sometimes medication	Informed consent
Epileptic seizures and myoclonus	Memory problems, embarrassment, personal safety, risk of injury, side effects of anticonvulsants	Anticonvulsants with evaluation of effect. Sometimes surgery	May have fluctuating capacity or temporary loss of capacity
Pain	Limits activity, lowers mood	Analgesia Non-invasive treatments, e.g. TENS, application of heat or cold. Distraction therapy, visualisation	Drug dosage and double effect
Respiratory problems	Chest infections, reduced activity, fatigue, low circulating oxygen levels	Posture and head position. Suctioning, medication for secretions, tracheostomy. Mechanical ventilation	Informed consent. Withholding, initiating and withdrawing treatment. Advance directives. Refusal of treatment

Nausea and vomiting	Malnutrition, loss of appetite, dehydration, electrolyte disturbance, mouth problems, feeling ill	Anti-emetics. Intravenous infusion. Artificial tube feeding. Nutritional assessment and mouth care	Withholding, initiating and withdrawing treatment. Advance directives
Fatigue	Limited activity and interaction	Paced activity with energy-sparing aids and equipment. Nutrition and oxygen level optimisation. Scheduled rest	
Bowel problems	Autonomic dysreflexia, triggering of spasticity, may contribute to nausea, loss of appetite, constipation, diarrhoea	Selective use of laxatives, bowel management programme to establish pattern. Stoma formation	Informed consent. Specialised training for some aspects of bowel management, e.g. manual evacuation
Urological problems	Autonomic dysreflexia, triggering of spasticity, disturbances of bladder storage and emptying	Fluid intake and output monitoring. Bladder triggering techniques. Intermittent catheterisation. Suprapubic and urethral catheterisation, oxybutinin	Informed consent
Psychiatric symptom and cognitive impairments	Inappropriate behaviour, fear, altered relationships, personal safety. Hallucinations, delusions, paranoia	Qualified assessment and management plan medication	Care and responsibility issues (previously Control and Restraint). Capacity to consent

transferred from a familiar care setting to an acute hospital environment. End-of-life issues for the patient arise, when and if the patient has expressed a wish about treatment and care options that would involve a change of care setting. Very often nurses are in a good position to support and care for the patient and family as death approaches and can facilitate the development of thorough care plans and not hesitate to call on the support of specialist professionals in the interdisciplinary team and other charities and support groups. In addition, for patients and nurses in a non-specialist setting there should be a link worker or outreach team who can help and advise on managing distressing discomforts.

LOSS AND GRIEF REACTIONS

Mourning is the time after bereavement or loss when grief is expressed. It may well be linked with religious observance and practices reflecting beliefs about life and death. Rituals help a grieving person to make sense of the experience within a socially accepted framework (Stewart 1992).

Grief is a normal reaction of intense sorrow involving physiological and psychological responses to loss of a person, a part of one's self or other aspect to which one is attached. *Anticipatory grieving* is the response to loss before it occurs.

Many patients and families will have already passed through cycles of anticipatory grieving as the disease has progressed. Anticipatory grieving has a host of emotional and behavioural manifestations. These may include:

- shock; numbness; denial; anger, despair and depression; guilt; blame; bargaining;
- altered activity, sleep disturbance, changed eating habits;
- fears are common about: pain and suffering; death and the process of dying; dying alone; beliefs about the afterlife and retribution; uncompleted tasks; loss and separation from family, friends and work; loss of personal dignity;
- easily fatigued, sighing, hyperventilation, feeling of lump in the throat.

This is similar to the normal process of actual grief once the loss has occurred and has been described by Accola and Albrecht

---

Box 14.2 Phases of grieving (Accola and Albrecht 1983)

1. **Impact**. Shock, numbness, unrealness, If anticipatory grieving has occurred, this phase may be shorter
2. **Disruption**. Numbness wears off, secondary losses of lifestyle relationships etc. become evident. Anger, depression, anxiety, exhaustion, impatience and cynicism may give rise to even more disturbing beliefs as person seeks to construct rationale and reasons for their suffering. May be difficult for others as it causes them discomfort. Person may be avoided for that reason.
3. **Recovery**. Suffering less intense although 'trigger events' such as birthdays and anniversaries cause strong grief reaction. These experiences can be helpful in moving the person on to the next stage.
4. **Growth**. People can demonstrate the positive results of their losses. Some may have spiritual renewal and speak of experiencing life more deeply.

(1983) in stages of impact, disruption, recovery and growth (see Box 14.2). The phases are not entirely sequential, may be cyclical and different members of a grieving family will be at different stages of the process. Sometimes grief may be dysfunctional, where reactions are inhibited, exaggerated, distorted or delayed. Such disturbance can interfere with normal function and cause mood swings, excessive crying, expressions of guilt and hopelessness, idealisation of the loss and developmental regression. In general care settings this can be difficult for a non-specialist to deal with, and if a family does seem to be in severe distress, help can be sought from specialists in the neurological field, counsellors or support groups.

LEGAL AND ETHICAL ASPECTS OF ARTIFICIAL HYDRATION AND NUTRITION

Legal and ethical issues of artificial hydration and nutrition are very complex and are mentioned here to raise awareness of that complexity. In 1993 the Law Lords allowed the nasogastric feeding of Tony Bland, who had been in a persistent vegetative state since the Hillsborough disaster in 1989, to be discontinued. The case provoked powerful emotions and a public perception that withdrawal of feeding meant starving someone to death (Tribe and Korgaonkar 1993; Lennard Jones 2000). Nurses are bound by the code of conduct to provide patients with the means of adequate nutrition and hydration, with an ethical duty to seek the patient's consent to initiate appropriate measures to monitor the effectiveness and maintain good nutrition (Scott 1999a,b; Shaw 2002; The *et al.* 2002).

Compassionate care to relieve distressing symptoms when a person is in the terminal phase of an illness may often involve the insertion of a tube in order to be able to administer nutrients and fluids compatible with sustaining life. The insertion of such a tube is regarded in law as a medical treatment as such the decision to carry out the procedure is based on the clinical judgement of the patient's best interests and on the informed consent of the patient (Sensky 2002). Refusal by the patient to allow the procedure to be carried out is binding and it would be ethically and legally wrong for a nurse to attempt to override this. However, that refusal must be the decision of someone with the capacity to make the decision (Gaul and Wilson 1990; Kent 1996; Baldwin and Hurley 2002).

Advance directives and living wills
There is a distinction between generalised and specific refusal of treatment. A patient's refusing a treatment close to the proposed intervention, at a time of full capacity, while suffering from the condition and with an understanding of the consequences of refusal is different from their making a general statement when they were not suffering from that condition. This needs to be considered when taking a person's wishes into account. The patient's mood when making the statement should also be considered, since stress or depression may temporarily cloud judgement (Lemke 2001). However, there is no legislation on advance directives.

CAPACITY TO GIVE INFORMED CONSENT
Sometimes it may be legal to enforce nutritional treatment on an unwilling patient with a mental disorder or on an *incompe-*

tent adult patient. The doctor undertaking care is responsible in law for the decision to give, withhold or withdraw medical treatment. For people to have the *capacity* to take a particular decision, they must be able both to

- comprehend and retain information material to the decision, especially as to the consequences of having or not having the intervention in question, and
- to use and weigh this information in the decision-making process.

Methods of assessing comprehension and ability to use information to make a choice include:

- exploring the patient's ability to paraphrase what has been said; (repeating and rewording explanations as necessary);
- exploring whether the patient is able to compare alternatives or to express any thoughts on possible consequences other than those that have been disclosed;
- exploring whether the patient applies the information to their own case.

Acting in the patient's best interests, doctors should enquire about the patient's previously expressed views, preferably in writing, about the type of treatment they would have wished under such circumstances. Although full consultation should be made with family, nurses and other members of the health care team (Lipley 1999), in English law relatives cannot take a decision on a behalf of a patient (Haddad 2000). The process and outcomes of the capacity to consent issue and treatment decision making should be documented.

PERSISTENT VEGETATIVE STATE

If the person is in a *persistent vegetative state* (see Box 13.1 in Chapter 13) an application to the court must be made to establish the legality of withdrawing nutrients given by tube, although the validity of this protocol has been questioned (Jennet 1999). For *incompetent patients* with conditions other than persistent vegetative state a protocol should be followed with every step documented. Sometimes an individual may feel uncomfortable with a decision to withdraw treatment (Ingham 2001). This is a matter of *conscience* and no nurse or carer must ever be expected to participate in an action or withdrawal of treatment that they believe to be morally wrong. Judges decide what is legal or illegal, which may be different from deciding what is morally right or wrong. Thus, once tube feeding was identified as medical treatment, withdrawal became a legal issue.

The decision to withdraw treatment is often based on expertise in the medical profession, by those who can make clinical judgements about a treatment's ability to preserve life, prevent disability, relieve pain and distress, and about the risks and burdens associated with treatment (Behi 1999) They are, however, no more competent than others in making judgements on non-clinical issues such as quality of life (Jarmulowicz 2001).

Quality of life

Quality of life and allocation of resources are often linked in making health care decisions. Bach and Barnett (1994) point out that quality of life is difficult if not impossible to measure by objective criteria that can be applied to all individuals. For this reason, decision making needs to take into account the patient's wishes, the family and culture to which they belong. Cultural and spiritual beliefs have a strong impact on end-of-life issues, the process of dying and the rituals at the time of death, funeral arrangements, mourning customs and beliefs about afterlife.

WITHDRAWING AND WITHHOLDING TREATMENT

There is a difference between *withdrawing* treatment and *withholding* it. Withholding is generally a medical decision, with consultation, often on the basis of biomedical futility. Once a treatment is initiated, patients have a legitimate right to continue the treatment unless they decide for themselves that they wish the treatment to discontinue. Thus tube feeding, once initiated, under current law cannot be withdrawn from patients who are in a persistent vegetative state without the intervention of the High Court. However, in the case of mechanical ventilation, the application of the *brain stem death criteria* will usually be the basis for the decision to withdraw ventilatory support.

Brain stem death criteria
The cranial nerves attach themselves to the brain stem and are a sensitive indicator of brain stem function. If all these reflexes are absent then the person is considered brain dead. A person who is brain dead is legally dead and there is no duty to continue to treat.

Brain stem death is indicated by:

- fixation of pupils;
- absence of corneal and vestibulo-occular reflexes;
- absence of response within the cranial nerve distribution to sensory stimuli;
- no response to bronchial stimulation when a catheter is passed into the trachea;
- no spontaneous breathing movement when the patient is disconnected from a mechanical ventilator. This apnoea test is the most conclusive that all brain stem function has ceased.

The condition should be present for 6–24 hours and requires confirmation by two experienced doctors on two separate occasions who are not assigned to the care of the patient and have not usually met the patient before taking the tests. Compassionate involvement of the family must be sensitively carried out and the full support of the care team given.

NURSING ASSESSMENT

The purpose of a nursing assessment is to recognise the needs, problems and wishes of patients and their families, the strengths and assets they already have as evidenced by their coping so far, and to ensure that provision is made for people to worship and express their religious beliefs. Not every nurse will feel comfortable addressing these important issues, but through an effective therapeutic relationship, assessment becomes possible, using techniques such as building rapport, reflective listening, open-ended questions, tolerance of pauses and silences, which will help elicit information and point the way to some suitable goals and interventions.

- How openly does the person express their thoughts, feelings and needs? A commonly used framework is that by Glaser and Strauss (1965) as shown in Box 14.3.

- How does this impact on ethical issues such as informed consent and end-of-life issues?
- What meaning does the loss or knowledge of the terminal stage of illness have for the patient and family and how is it affecting their lives and relationships?
- Are there cultural aspects and beliefs which the care team need to know about?
- What coping skills has the patient already demonstrated and how does their mood or condition affect their energy levels?
- Are the patient's physical discomforts exacerbated by psychological or spiritual distress?
- Is the family supportive and are their interrelationships open and trusting?
- Is it appropriate to contact other members of the care team or to suggest other support mechanisms?

Box 14.3 Levels of awareness in terminal illness (Glaser and Strauss 1965)

Closed awareness
This is similar to denial in so far as the patient does not recognise the terminal nature of the illness.

Suspicion awareness
The patient suspects that others know something that they are not telling them and employs strategies to try to confirm or refute the suspicion.

Mutual pretence awareness
Patient, family and staff realise that the person is dying but all pretend that the other does not know.

Open awareness
Patient, family and staff recognise and accept that the person is dying and they act on this awareness relatively openly.

INTERVENTIONS

- Meet the trust and security needs of the patient and family first. This may not be wholly met by nurses, but nurses are in a position to contact sources of support if they have developed a therapeutic relationship with the patient and family.
- Ensure that interaction with the patient and the use of aids and equipment enhance dignity and self-esteem, as the patient or the patient's family perceive them.
- Assess and alleviate physical discomforts, for example those shown in Table 14.1.
- In the early stages of grieving, allow protective numbness but avoid reinforcing denial.
- Be available and accept without judgement the thoughts and emotions the person expresses. Ask: What needs to be done? How can I help?
- Acknowledge depth of feelings and help label feelings, for example: Does that make you feel angry? Be prepared for anger to be directed at the care team or care setting. Begin to explore implications of the loss or anticipated loss and what small steps might help towards recovery. Explore potential of routines and what events trigger strong emotional reactions.
- As the therapeutic relationship evolves it may be possible to move from non-directive to more active helping approaches. Constantly reassess physical, psychosocial and spiritual well-being.
- Help the patient increase awareness of the available support, such as family, support groups and other professionals, and to recognise their own coping skills, strengths and capabilities.
- As the relationship becomes more open, recognise the progress the patient has made in taking opportunities for growth. Accept that the patient may have resolved some dilemmas they had about end-of-life issues.

ROLE OF THE NURSE

As with other situations that are difficult to face, individual nurses may have different levels of confidence and expertise in planning care. However, all nurses have a responsibility to recognise distress in palliative and terminal stage of illness

(Hickey 1997) and to provide sensitive care in assessing, planning, implementing and evaluating nursing care.

They can help orientate the patient and family to the care setting and services available, liaising with the family spokesperson and regularly updating them on the patient's condition or progress. They can seek information from the family about the patient's preferences and support the family in the grieving process. The nurse is also responsible for recognising the need for referral to other professionals or to voluntary support resources. The nursing care plan is therefore a key document and should record details of the support and information given, other interventions, and patient or family responses.

SUMMARY
❏ Palliative care for people with progressive neurological disease often takes place in non-specialist community, hospital and care home settings. The service can be improved by specialist link workers and outreach teams offering support in neurological palliative care.
❏ Effective listening, appropriate referrals and giving information about care and professional support can help patients and families at the various stages in the grieving process.
❏ End-of-life issues that arise in neurological care include aspects of informed consent, capacity to give consent, refusal of treatment, request not to initiate a treatment, and the withdrawal of a treatment such as mechanical ventilation or nutritional support and hydration via a tube.
❏ Nurses have the responsibility for recognising the ethical and legal aspects of the activities and interventions in palliative care, for ensuring relief of physical and mental suffering and contacting specialist help when needed.

REFERENCES
Accola, K. M. and Albrecht, M. (1983) Loss and grieving. In Snyder, M. (ed.) *A Guide to Neurological and Neurosurgical Nursing*, John Wiley, New York, Chapter 17.
Axford, J. and O'Callaghan, C. (2004) *Medicine*, 2nd edn. Blackwell, Oxford.

Bach, J. R. and Barnett, V. (1994) Ethical considerations in the management of individuals with severe neuromuscular disorders. *American Journal of Medical Rehabilitation* **73**, 134–40.

Baldwin, A. and Hurley, C. (2002) Assisting death or letting die? Withdrawing treatment at the patient's request. *Nursing in Critical Care* **7** (5), 241–6.

Behi, R. H. (1999) Witholding nutrition and hydration: 'Nutrition and hydration are not options but rights'. *British Journal of Nursing* **8** (14), 916.

BMA (n.d.) http://www.bma.org.uk/ap.nsf/Content/pas+project +discussions+definitions

Chapman, C. R. and Gavrin, J. (1995) Suffering and the dying patient. *Journal of Pharmaceutical Care in Pain and Symptom Control* **3** (3/4), 67–90.

Gaul, A. L. and Wilson, S. E. (1990) Should a ventilator be removed at a patient's request? *Journal of Neuroscience Nursing* **22** (5), 326–9.

Glaser, B. E. and Strauss, A. L. (1965) *Awareness of Dying*. Aldine, New York.

Haddad, A. (2000) Acute care decisions. Ethics in action . . . family of a comatose ventilator dependent patient insists that all forms of treatment be continued. *Registered Nurse* **63** (9), 25–8, 101.

Hickey, J. (1997) *The Clinical Practice of Neurological and Neurosurgical Nursing*, 4th edn. Lippincott, New York.

Ingham, J. (2001) Nurses' perceptions relating to withholding and withdrawing of life prolonging treatments. *Nursing in Critical Care* **6** (4), 171–4.

Jarmulowicz, M. (2001) Submission to the GMC on withholding and withdrawing life prolonging treatments: good practice in decision making. *Joint Ethico-Medical Committee of the Catholic Union of Great Britain and the Guild of Catholic Doctors*, available at http:// www.catholicdoctors.org.uk/submissions/GMC

Jennet, B. (1999) Should cases of permanent vegetative state still go court? Britain should follow other countries and keep the courts for cases of dispute. *British Medical Journal* **319** (7213), 796–7.

Kent, M. A. (1996) The ethical arguments concerning the artificial ventilation of patients with motor neurone disease. *Nursing Ethics: an International Journal for Health Care Professionals* **3** (4), 317–28.

Lemke, D. M. (2001) Patient requested removal of ventilatory support in high level tetraplegai: guidelines for the health provider. *SCI Nursing* **18** (2), 67–73.

Lennard Jones, J. (2000) Legal and ethical aspects of feeding. *NT Plus* **96** (17), 7.

Lipley, N. (1999) Nurses must be consulted over end of life decisions. *Nursing Standard* **8** (7), 412.

Neurological Alliance (2001a) *In Search of a Service*. Neurological Alliance London.

Neurological Alliance (2001b) *Levelling Up Standards of Care for People with a Neurological Condition.* Neurological Alliance, London.

Scott, H. (1999a) Nurse must protect patients nutritional rights. *British Journal of Nursing* **8** (7), 412.

Scott, H. (1999b) Nutrition and hydration are not options but rights. *British Journal of Nursing* **8** (13), 842.

Sensky, T. (2002) Withdrawal of life sustaining treatment: patient autonomy and values conflict with the responsibilities of clinicians. *British Medical Journal* **325** (7357), 175–6.

Shaw, S. (2002) Legal issues surrounding consent and withdrawing and withholding treatment: a case study. *Nursing in Critical Care* **7** (2), 94–8.

Stewart, W. (1992) *An A–Z of Counselling Theory and Practice.* Chapman & Hall, London.

The, A., Pasman, R., Onwuteaka-Philipsen, B., Ribble, M. and van der Wal, G. (2002) Withholding the artificial administration of fluids and food from elderly patients with dementia: ethnographic study. *British Medical Journal* **325** (7376), 1326–9.

Tribe, D. and Korgaonkar, G. (1993) Ethical and legal. Withdrawing medical treatment: implications of the Bland case. *British Journal of Nursing* **2** (1), 84–6.

National Service Framework for Long Term Conditions and Skill Competencies in Neurological Care

15

In a practical handbook such as this there is not the scope to address care management systems, structures and services that can provide ready access to specialist help and advice, integrate care into pathways and implement the standards set by the National Service Framework for Long Term Conditions (Department of Health, 2004).

The National Service Framework (NSF) aims to make sure that services for people with long-term neurological conditions and their families and carers are:

- quicker and easier to use;
- more closely matched to people's needs;
- better co-ordinated – so people do not have to see too many professionals and tell them the same information about themselves again and again;
- provided for as long as people need them, so that treatment continues without the need for a new referral every time the person has a new problem;
- better at helping people with neurological conditions and their carers to make decisions about care and treatment;
- provided by people with knowledge and experience of specific conditions;
- giving people with long-term neurological conditions better results from their treatment;
- planned around the views of people with long-term neurological conditions and their carers;

- able to give people more choice about how and where they get treatment and care;
- better at helping people to live more independently

1. A person-centred service

This is a main theme that runs throughout the NSF. All people with long-term neurological conditions are offered a full assessment of their health and social care needs. In addition, they are to be offered information and education about their condition; the chance to make decisions about their treatment; and to be involved in writing a plan about how their needs will be met (a care plan).

2. Early recognition followed by prompt diagnosis and treatment

Anyone suspected of having a long-term neurological condition is to quickly see a doctor or other professional with expert knowledge of that condition. They should have tests, be given a diagnosis and have any treatment they need. This should be as close to home as possible. This is so that a correct diagnosis and appropriate treatment happens as soon as possible.

3. Emergency and acute management

Anyone admitted to hospital for a neurosurgical or neurological emergency is assessed and treated by professionals with the right skills and experience who have access to the right facilities and equipment.

4. Early and specialist rehabilitation

Anyone with a long-term neurological condition who would benefit from rehabilitation is to receive timely, high quality rehabilitation services in hospital or other specialist settings when they need them. When ready, they are to receive the support they need to return home for more community rehabilitation and support.

5. Community rehabilitation and support

People with long-term neurological conditions living at home are to receive a full range of rehabilitation, advice and support to meet their continuing and changing needs. This is to increase their independence and help them to live as they wish.

6. Vocational rehabilitation

People with long-term neurological conditions are to have appropriate support to help them find or regain employment, to remain in work or to pursue educational opportunities.

7. Equipment and accommodation

People with long-term neurological conditions are to have the equipment they need (such as wheelchairs), within an appropriate timeframe and to have adaptations made to their homes as and when needed, to support them to live independently; help them with their care; maintain their health; and improve their quality of life.

8. Personal care and support

Health and social care services are to work together to ensure that people with long-term neurological conditions are given the care and support they need to live independently in their own homes wherever possible.

9. Palliative care

People with long-term neurological conditions nearing the end of their life are to have access to a range of palliative care services as and when they need them, to control symptoms and offer pain relief, and to meet any personal needs they may have.

10. Support for family and carers

All carers of people with long-term neurological conditions are to receive appropriate support and services which recognise their needs as a carer and as an individual in their own right.

11. Care during admission to hospital or other health and social care settings

All people with long-term neurological conditions are to have their specific neurological needs met when they are receiving care for any other reason in any health or social care setting.

Among the recommendations for early action to help organisations prepare for and start implementing the NSF is the need to analyse and profile the skills of the local workforce. See Skills for Health long term neurological conditions project at http://www.skillsforhealth.org.uk/content/project.php?p=53. These skills are likely to include the following:

- Develop relationships with individuals with neurological conditions.
- Communicate with individuals with neurological conditions.
- Provide information to individuals with neurological conditions.
- Enable individuals to manage their neurological condition.
- Provide information and support to carers of individuals with neurological condition.
- Refer individuals with neurological conditions.
- Respond to referrals of individuals with neurological conditions.
- Assess the condition of individuals with neurological conditions.
- Conduct clinical examinations of individuals with neurological conditions.
- Propose a diagnosis of a neurological condition.
- Agree and plan the provision of interventions for managing neurological conditions.
- Co-ordinate the care of individuals with neurological conditions.
- Provide interventions to individuals with neurological conditions.
- Enable individuals with neurological conditions to manage their symptoms.
- Enable individuals to manage changes in their neurological conditions.
- Enable individuals with neurological conditions to respond to acute episodes.
- Support individuals with neurological conditions to manage their medication.
- Support individuals with neurological conditions to manage their respiratory function.

- Support individuals with neurological conditions to manage their nutrition.
- Support individuals with neurological conditions to optimise their physical functions.
- Support individuals with neurological conditions to optimise their psychological functions.
- Support individuals with neurological conditions to optimise their communication skills.
- Support individuals with neurological conditions to optimise their independence.

Appendix 2 to this book provides a list of suggested further reading and other resources that give more detailed and thorough guidance in the many aspects of neurological nursing.

Appendix 1
Resources and Support Groups

Ataxia UK
10 Winchester House
Kennington Park
Cranmer Road
London
SW9 6EJ
T: 0207 582 9444
F: 0207 582 1444
E: enquiries@ataxia.org.uk
W: http://www.ataxia.org.uk/
Conducts fundraising to support medical research into causes and potential therapies. Provides information, advice and support to people affected by ataxia.

BASIC (Brain and Spinal Injuries Charity)
The Neurocare Centre
554 Eccles New Road
Salford
M5 2AL
T: 0161 787 4558
F: 0161 707 6441
E: Enquiries@basiccharity.org.uk
W: http://www.basiccharity.org.uk/
Provides information and support for people affected by neurological conditions. Runs a number of self-help groups around the UK. Promotes research into neurological conditions.

Brain and Spine Foundation
7 Winchester House
Kennington Park
Cranmer Road

London
SW9 6EJ
T: 020 7793 5900
Brain and Spine Helpline: 0808 808 1000
F: 020 7793 5939
E: info@brainandspine.org.uk
W: http://www.brainandspine.org.uk/
Aims to improve the quality of life for people with neurological disorders and to reduce neurological disability through research, education, and patient and carer support and information programmes.

Epilepsy Action
New Anstey House
Gate Way Drive
Yeadon
Leeds
LS19 7XY
T: 0113 210 8800
Helpline 0808 800 5050
F: 0113 391 0300
E: info@epilepsy.org.uk
W: http://www.epilepsy.org.uk/
Provides advice and information services for people with epilepsy, their families and those who care for them. Also campaigns for improved health and social services.

Guillain-Barré Syndrome Support Group
Lincolnshire County Council Offices
Eastgate
Sleaford
Lincolnshire
NG34 7EB
T: 01529 304615
F: 01529 304 615
E: admin@gbs.org.uk
W: http://www.gbs.org.uk/
Provides emotional support to sufferers of GBS, CIDP and related conditions, and their families. Provides literature to suf-

ferers, families, medical professionals. Educates public and medical community about the Support Group and maintains awareness of the illness. Fosters research.

Headway – The Brain Injury Association
2 Tavistock Place
London
WC1H 9RA
T: 0207 841 0241
F: 0207 841 0240
E: info@headway.org.uk
W: http://www.headway.org.uk/
Supports people with brain injury, their families and carers, and concerned professionals. Has 115 groups throughout the UK, 57 of which run activity/rehabilitation centres called Headway Houses. Campaigns for improved statutory services for people with brain injury.

HemiHelp
Unit 1
Wellington Works
Wellington Road
London
SW19 8EQ
T: 0845 120 3713
Helpline: 0845 123 2372 (Mon–Fri 10.00am–1pm)
F: 0845 120 3723
E: helpline@hemihelp.org.uk
W: http://www.hemihelp.org.uk/
Provides information and support for children with hemiplegia (acquired and congenital) and aims to increase public and professional awareness of hemiplegia and its associated conditions.

Joint Epilepsy Council
PO Box 186
Leeds
LS20 8NH
T: 01943 871 852
E: sharon.jec@btconnect.com

W: http://www.jointepilepsycouncil.org.uk/
An umbrella organisation that exists to enable epilepsy organisations to work together for the benefit of people who have epilepsy.

Meningitis Trust
Fern House
Bath Road
Stroud
GL5 3TJ
T: 01453 768000
Helpline 0845 6000 800 (24-hours, nurse-led)
F: 01453 768001
Textphone: 01453 768003
E: info@meningitis-trust.org
E: helpline@meningitis-trust.org
W: http://www.meningitis-trust.org/
Supports individuals, families and communities, and produces an extensive range of information to raise awareness about meningitis and meningococcal septicaemia. Invests in research programmes and also provides education for health care professionals. Provides financial grants, a national counselling and home visits service to those affected by meningitis and/or meningococcal septicaemia.

Motor Neurone Disease Association
PO Box 246
Northampton
NN1 2PR
T: 01604 250505
F: 01604 638289
E: info@mndassociation.org
W: http://www.mndassociation.org/
Works to ensure that people affected by MND secure the highest standards of care in order to achieve quality of life. Stimulates and funds research into the causes of MND. Provides a helpline, information, equipment loan, financial support, a network of regional care advisers, local branches and volunteer visitors.

Multiple Sclerosis Society
Ms National Centre
372 Edgware Road
Cricklewood
London
NW2 6ND
T: 020 8438 0701
F: 020 8438 0700
E: info@mssociety.org.uk
W: http://www.mssociety.org.uk/
Provides support and information for people affected by MS through a network of branches (about 370 around the UK) and through helpline and publications. Carries out research into MS and policy work and campaigns on MS issues. Also provides respite and holiday homes.

Multiple Sclerosis Trust
Spirella Building
Bridge Road
Letchworth
Herts
SG6 4ET
T: 01462 476710
F: 01462 476700
E: info@mstrust.org.uk
W: http://www.mstrust.org.uk/
A leading UK charity for people with MS, their families and friends, and for the health and social care professionals who work with them. Offers practical, deliverable solutions, including: information about MS which is positive and constructive; education for nurses and other professionals; research which is relevant to people who live with MS; and support for MS specialist nurses.

National Society for Epilepsy
Chesham Lane
Chalfont St Peter
Bucks
SL9 0RJ

T: 01494 871927
F: 01494 601300
E: info@epilepsynse.org.uk
W: http://www.epilepsynse.org.uk/
Seeks to enhance the health and well-being of people with
epilepsy by improving clinical treatment and care and by the
provision of health information to people with epilepsy, to
health professionals and the general public.

Parkinson's Disease Society
215 Vauxhall Bridge Road
London
SW1V 1EJ
T: 0207 932 1351
E: info@parkinsons.org.uk
W: http://www.parkinsons.org.uk/
Provides practical support, information and advice to people
with Parkinson's disease and their carers. Funds research to
investigate the causes of Parkinson's disease, to improve the
treatments available and to develop new treatment techniques.

Speakability
1 Royal Street
London
SE1 7LL
T: 020 7261 9572
F: 020 7261 9542
E: speakability@speakability.org.uk
W: http://www.speakability.org.uk/
Supports people with aphasia, and those that care for them,
through its information service and network of self-help groups.
Campaigns to increase awareness of aphasia as a long-term con-
dition. Provides training to paid and unpaid carers on commu-
nication skills.

The Stroke Association
Stroke House
240 City Road
London

EC1V 2PR
T: 020 7490 2686
E: info@stroke.org.uk
W: http://www.stroke.org.uk/
Aims to help all in England and Wales affected by stroke. Develops and provides services, supports research, disseminates knowledge, provides training and education to improve standards of care.

UK Acquired Brain Injury Forum (UKABIF)
Royal Hospital for Neurodisability
West Hill
Putney
London SW15 3SW
T: 0208 780 4569
E: ukabif@rhn.org.uk
W: http://www.ukabif.org.uk/
A not-for-profit coalition of organisations and individuals that seek to promote understanding of all aspects of acquired brain injury (ABI) and provide information and expert input to policy makers and others to promote the interests of brain-injured people and their families. Encourages the development of good practice by setting up working parties and conferences to discuss any aspect of ABI and supports the All Party Parliamentary Group on Acquired Brain Injury.

Appendix 2
Further Reading

Burgess, M. (2002) *Multiple Sclerosis Theory and Practice for Nurses.* Whurr, London.

Department of Health (2005) *National Service Framework for Long Term Conditions.* HMSO, London.

Edwards, S. (2002) *Neurological Physiotherapy*, 2nd edn. Churchill Livingstone, Edinburgh.

Grieve, J. (1999) *Neuropsychology for Occupational Therapists*, 2nd edn. Blackwell, Oxford.

Holland, K., Jenkins, J., Solomon, J. and Whittam, S. (2003) *Applying the Roper, Logan and Tierney Model in Practice.* Churchill Livingstone, Edinburgh.

Hickey, J. (1997) *The Clinical Practice of Neurological and Neurosurgical Nursing*, 4th edn. Lippincott, New York.

Multiple Sclerosis Trust (2000) *Multiple Sclerosis Information for Health and Social Care Professionals.* Multiple Sclerosis Trust, Letchworth.

National Institute for Clinical Excellence (2003) *Head Injury Guidelines*, CG4, available at http://www.nice.org.uk

National Institute for Clinical Excellence (2003) *Multiple Sclerosis Management of Multiple Sclerosis in Primary and Secondary Care*, CG8, available at http://www.nice.org.uk

National Institute for Clinical Excellence (2004) *The Diagnosis and Care of Children and Adults with Epilepsy*, CG020, available at http://www.nice.org.uk

National Institute for Clinical Excellence (2004) *Falls: The Assessment and Prevention of Falls in Older People*, CG21, available at http://www.nice.org.uk

Neurological Alliance (2001) *Levelling Up Standards of Care for People with a Neurological Condition.* Neurological Alliance, London.

Pound, C., Parr, S., Lindsay, J. and Woolf, C. (2000) *Beyond Aphasia: Therapies for Living with Communication Disability.* Winslow Press, Bicester.

Royal College of Physicians (1999) *National Clinical Guidelines for Stroke.* The Intercollgiate Working Party for Stroke. National Electronic Library for Health, available at http://www.nelh.nhs.uk/guidelinesdb/html/stroke-ft.htm

Royal College of Physicians (2002) *National Clinical Guidelines for Stroke: Update 2002*. The Intercollegiate Working Party for Stroke, Royal College of Physicians, London.

Shorvon, S. and Walker, M. (2000) *MIMS Guide to Epilepsy*, 2nd edn. Glaxo Wellcome, Uxbridge.

Stewart-Amidei, C. and Kunkel, J. A. (2001) *AANN's Neuroscience Nursing: Human Responses to Neurologic Dysfunction*, 2nd edn. W. B. Saunders, New York.

Weiner, H. L., Levitt, L. P. and Rae-Grant, A. (2004) *Neurology*, 7th edn. Lippincott, Williams & Wilkins, New York.

Wilson, B. A. and McLellan, D. L. (eds) (19997) *Rehabilitation Studies Handbook*. Cambridge University Press, Cambridge.

Index

acoustic nerve damage, 223
action potential, 8
advance statements (directives),
    274, 280
agitation, 80, 81–2
agnosia, 46, 234, 236
airway secretions, 110, 117
    nursing interventions, 110–12,
    120
    suctioning, 111–15
allodynia, 44, 55–6
analgesics, 53
anticholinergic drugs, 162, 163
aphasia, 20, 89, 92, 93, 276
    assessment, 93–100
    GCS scoring, 36, 37
    types, 94
apraxia, 20, 46, 177
    oral, 92–3
ataxia, 42, 43, 218, 223
autonomic dysfunction, 24, 194–5
autonomic dysreflexia, 24, 163–4,
    195
autonomic nerves, 2, 5, 23, 192

baclofen, 205, 206
balance, 42–3, 204
bathing equipment, 178–85, 187
bed rails, 74, 76
beds, 211–12, 220
bedwetting, 163
behaviour, 23–5
bladder, 154, 155
    compression/triggering, 161

dysfunction, *see* neurogenic
    bladder
    retraining, 158–60
    washouts, 159
blood–brain barrier, 18
blood pressure (BP), 31–2, 223
body image deficits, 177, 234,
    235
body scheme deficits, 234, 235
botulinum toxin, 207–208
bowel problems, 166–73, 277
    interventions (retraining),
    170–71
    nursing assessment, 168–9
bowel storage/evacuation, 156,
    166–8
brain, 4, 14–19
    functional areas, 14–17
    protection, 17–19
    tumours, 169
brain injury
    communication problems, 90,
    100
    elimination problems, 167, 169
    mobility problems, 205,
    207–208, 218
    respiratory problems, 109, 120
    sleeping problems, 266, 269
    temperature control problems,
    194, 195, 198–9
    washing/dressing problems,
    180
brain stem death criteria, 282–3
brain tumours, 273

breathing, 105–23
breath sounds, 110

casts, 210, 221
catheterisation, urinary, 158–9,
    161–2
central nervous system, 2, 3
cerebrospinal fluid, 17
chairs, 215, 216, 221, 222
chest infections, 105, 110, 120, 195
children, 243
circle of Willis, 17
clothing, adaptive, 186
cognitive deficits, 46–7, 72–4, 178,
    231–4, 277
cognitive processing, 14, 15
communication, 86–104
    assessment, 47, 93–100
    facilitating, 98–9
    problems, 89–90, 91–3
confusion, 72–4
consciousness
    assessment, 33–8
    causes of impaired, 34, 263,
        264–6
consent, capacity to give, 280–81
constipation, 163, 169
contraception, 252
contractures, 69, 205–206
co-ordination, assessment, 42–3
cough, 111, 127
counselling, 251
cranial nerves, 19, 21, 22, 40
critical-illness neuropathy, 22, 217
cushions, 213

death, brain stem, 282–3
defecation, 156, 166–8
delirium, 12
dementia, 20, 25
    communication problems, 90
    eating and drinking problems,
        128

elimination problems, 167, 169
    respiratory problems, 109
    safety problems, 66, 67, 73–4
    washing/dressing problems,
        180
dental hygiene, 135, 178, 185–6
deodorants, 186
depression, 238, 239–41
desmopressin, 163
detrusor areflexia, 159, 162–3
detrusor hyperreflexia, 159, 162,
    163
detrusor muscle, 154
detrusor-sphincter dyssynergia,
    154, 159
dieticians, 143–4
disability, 229, 230, 242–3, 244–5
    see also mobility problems
disinhibited behaviours, 253–5
disorientation, 81, 178
double effect, 275
dressing, see washing and
    dressing
drinking, 124–52
driving, 245–6
drooling, 117–18
drugs
    enterally fed patients, 147–50
    side effects, 67, 158, 169, 238,
        250–51
dying, 272–88
dysarthria, 20, 91–3, 99, 276
dysautonomia, 194–5
dysphagia, 131–2, 142, 276
    feeding techniques, 137–8,
        139–40
    management, 141
dysphasia, 93

eating, 124–52
electrolytes, 7–8, 11–12
elimination, 153–75
end-of-life issues, 279–83

enteral nutrition, 138–50
    drug administration, 147–9
    mouth care, 144–7
    professional/ethical issues, 150, 279–82
    trouble shooting, 143–4, 145–6
epilepsy, 260–64
    drug side-effects, 66, 67, 90
    eating and drinking problems, 128
    washing/dressing problems, 180
erectile dysfunction, 250, 251
ethical issues, 78–9, 150, 279–83
euthanasia, 275

faecal incontinence, 169, 170–71
falls
    prevention, 78–9
    risk assessment, 74–8
    risk factors, 65–9, 72–4
family
    impact of illness, 242–3
    terminally ill patients, 278–9, 281, 286
fatigue, 126, 236–9, 277
feeding
    aids and equipment, 135, 136
    assistance, 133–5, 136–8
    techniques, 137–8, 139–40
fever, 191, 192–3, 197–8
food
    consistency, 140, 142
    serving, 133–5, 136
footwear, 186

gag reflex, 127
gait, 43
gastrostomy feeding, 143
Glasgow Coma Scale (GCS), 3, 34–8
grief reactions, 278–9
grooming aids/equipment, 185–6

Guillain-Barré syndrome (GBS), 23, 24, 63, 109, 194

hair care, 179, 185
handling, patient, 211, 214, 222
headache, 63
hemiplegia, 208–209, 223–4
hoists, 214
humidification, 116–17
hyperalgesia, 56
hyperpyrexia, 192–3
hypersexuality, 253–5
hyperthermia, 194
hypothermia, 193–4, 198

immobility, 68–9
infections, 195, 197–8, 238
inhibitory positions, 204, 221
injuries
    prevention, 78–9
    risk assessment, 74–8
    risk factors, 65–9, 72–4
insomnia, 259, 267, 268
intracranial pressure, raised, 31–2, 33
investigations, 47, 48

jejunostomy feeding, 143

language, 87–93
    assessment, 95–6
    see also aphasia
laxatives, 171, 172
legal issues, 78–9, 279–83
leisure activities, 244
libido, loss of, 250–51
living wills, 280
locked-in syndrome, 264
loss, 278–9
low awareness states, 265–6

malnutrition, 124, 126–7
mattresses, 211–12, 220

menstruation, 252
micturition, 154, 155
mobility aids and equipment,
    211–17
mobility problems, 201–28
    interventions, 220–24
    nursing assessment, 217–20
mood, 23–5, 230
motivation, 230
motor ability
    altered, 66, 68–9, 177, 205–24
    assessment, 40–43, 209
motor neurone disease, 10
    communication problems, 88,
        90, 91–3
    eating and drinking problems,
        128, 150
    fatigue, 239
    mobility problems, 217
    respiratory problems, 109,
        119–20
motor pathways, 3, 12, 13
motor processing, 14, 15
mourning, 278
mouth care, 144–7
movements, 202–205
    compensatory, 204
    repetitive, 69, 80–81
    voluntary/involuntary, 6
multiple sclerosis, 8, 10
    communication problems, 89,
        91–3
    depression, 239–40, 241
    eating and drinking problems,
        128
    elimination problems, 162–3,
        167, 169
    fatigue, 236–8, 239
    impact on family, 242–3
    mobility problems, 218
    respiratory problems, 109
    safety problems, 63, 66, 67, 72
    sexuality problems, 249, 252

    temperature control problems,
        194, 195
    washing/dressing problems,
        180
muscle
    innervation, 204
    power, assessment, 40–41
    tone, 69, 202–204, 222
    weakness, 217, 218
myelin, 8

nail care, 178, 185
nasogastric/nasojejunal/
        nasoduodenal feeding, 143
National Service Framework for
        Long Term Conditions,
        289–93
nausea and vomiting, 277
nerve impulse conduction, 7–8, 9
nervous system, 2–12
neuritis, 8
neurogenic bladder, 154–66, 167,
        195
    interventions, 158–63, 164–6
    nursing assessment, 157–8
    psychosocial effects, 171–2
    types, 159
neurogenic bowel, uninhibited,
        169
neuroglial cells, 18
neurological assessment, 33–43
neurones, 6–7
    disturbances of function, 11–12
    function, 7–8, 9
    organisation and integration,
        12–14
neuropathic pain, 8, 55–7
neuropathies, 8, 22–3
neurotransmission, 9, 10–11
neurotransmitters, 3–5, 10
nocturia, 163
non-treatment, 274–5
nursing assessment, 28–51

nutrition, 124–52
  assessment, 132–3, 134
  care planning, 132–3
  enteral, *see* enteral nutrition
  factors affecting, 125–6
  national guidelines, 131

observations, general, 30–33
occupational therapy, 230–31,
    234–6
  assessment, 45–6, 231
  communication problems,
    100
  mobility problems, 210, 218
  respiratory problems, 119
  self-care difficulties, 186–7
oral hygiene, 135, 144–7, 178,
    185–6
overflow incontinence, 156, 157,
    158

padding, 213, 220
pain, 53–65, 66, 276
  acute/chronic, 53–5
  assessment, 58–64
  descriptors, 56
  gate control theory, 64
  management, 53, 54, 64–5
  neuropathic, 8, 55–7
  nociceptive, 55, 56
  non-verbal indicators, 62
  psychosomatic (psychogenic),
    57
palliative care, 272, 273–8, 291
parallel processing, 15
parasomnia, 259, 268
parasympathetic nerves, 5, 23
Parkinson's disease, 10, 11
  communication problems, 88,
    89, 91–3
  depression, 241
  eating and drinking problems,
    128

elimination problems, 167, 173
mobility problems, 216–17,
    218
safety problems, 66, 67, 68
sexual dysfunction, 250
sleep problems, 268
washing/dressing problems,
    180
pelvic floor exercises, 160, 171
perceptual deficits, 66, 72–4, 177,
    234–6
perceptual processing, 14
peripheral nervous system, 2, 3,
    19–22
  problems, 22–3, 24
peripheral neuropathy, 22–3
persistent vegetative state, 109,
    264, 265, 279–80, 281–2
personality, 23–5
pharmacist, 144, 147, 148
phonation, 87–93
physiotherapy, 43–4, 118–19,
    209–10
P-LI-SS-IT model, 252, 254
postural tone, 202–204
posture, abnormal, 202, 203,
    204
pregnancy, 252
pressure sores, 65–6
  prevention, 66
  risk assessment, 70, 71
  risk factors, 65–9
proprioception, 68, 204–205
psychiatric symptoms, 277
psychological assessment, 47–9
psychosocial problems, 171–2,
    188–9, 230, 249
psychotherapy, 241
pulse, 31
pulse oximetry, 31, 111
pupillary responses, 39–40

quality of life, 243–4, 282

reflexes, 6, 15, 41–2
respiration
    assessment, 31, 108–10, 115
    mechanisms, 106–108
    problems, 108–10, 118–20, 276
restlessness, 69, 75, 80–81
restraint, 78–9
reticular activating system (RAS),
    33

safe environment, maintaining,
    52–85
saliva, drooling, 117–18
seating, 214–15, 221, 222
sedation, 82
seizures, 260–64, 268, 276
    driving and, 245–6
    symptoms, 69, 74, 75, 80–81,
    263
self-care activities, see washing
    and dressing
sensory assessment, 44–5
sensory disturbances, 44–5, 66,
    67–8, 177
sensory overload, 80
sensory pathways, 2–3, 13
sensory processing, 14, 15
serial processing, 15
sexual dysfunction, 249–51,
    252–3, 254
sexuality, expressing, 248–56
sexually disinhibited behaviour,
    253–5
shaving, 185
sheets, low friction (slide), 212–13
showering equipment, 178–85,
    187
sitting balance, 204
sleep, 257–71
    apnoea, 259, 268
    deprivation, 259–60
    disturbances, 238, 257–71
    stages and states, 258

somnolence, excessive, 259
spasms, 204, 205
spasticity, 12, 198–9, 205–208, 276
spatial relations deficit, 177–8,
    234, 235
speech, 87–93
    articulation problems, see
    dysarthria
    assessment, 95–6
speech and language therapy, 47,
    96–100, 119, 143–4, 147
spinal cord, 19
spinal cord injury, 63, 109, 163–4,
    169
spinal nerves, 19, 22
splinting, 210, 221
steroid therapy, 195
stress incontinence, 156, 158, 164
stroke, 17, 20
    communication problems, 89,
    100–101
    depression, 241
    eating and drinking problems,
    128, 132, 135–7
    elimination problems, 166, 167
    mobilising problems, 208–209
    respiratory problems, 109
    safety problems, 56, 57, 63, 66,
    67
    sexual dysfunction, 249, 250
    sleep disturbances, 259
    washing/dressing problems,
    180
subarachnoid haemorrhage, 11,
    63
suctioning, airway, 111–15
suicide, 240
swallowing
    assessment, 47, 129, 130, 132
    difficulty, see dysphagia
    mechanism, 127–9
sympathetic nerves, 5, 23
synapses, 10–11

temperature (body), 32–3,
191–200
control mechanisms, 192–4
disturbed control, 194–5, 223
measurement, 195–6
nursing assessment, 196–7
temperature (environmental)
hypersensitivity, 194, 195, 196,
198–9
hyposensitivity, 194, 195, 196–7
terminal care, 272, 273–8
terminal illness, 274, 279–86
interventions, 285
legal and ethical issues, 279–83
nursing assessment, 283–4
tests, diagnostic, 47, 48
tracheostomy, 115–17, 119
transport, 245–6
traumatic brain injury
eating and drinking problems,
128
mobility problems, 207–208,
221–4
rehabilitation, 245
safety problems, 63, 66
sexual dysfunction, 251
sleeping problems, 259
treatment
refusal, 274, 280
withdrawing/withholding,
274–5, 279–80, 282–3
T-rolls, 212, 220
tube feeding, see enteral nutrition

urge incontinence, 156, 157, 158
urinary incontinence, 156, 157–66,
167
urinary problems, 154–66, 277
urinary tract infections, 157, 195
urine
collection/storage devices,
164–6
residual, 157
storage and voiding, 154, 155
utensils, special, 135, 136

vegetative state, 264
persistent, see persistent
vegetative state
ventilation, mechanical, 119, 282
visual impairment, 68, 73, 224
voiding, 154, 155
vomiting, 277

walking, 223
walking aids, 215
wandering, 72–3, 74, 79, 81, 198
washing and dressing, 176–90
aids and equipment, 179–86
assessment, 186–7
interventions, 179, 187–8
wheelchairs, 214–15
work, 244–5
working and playing, 229–47